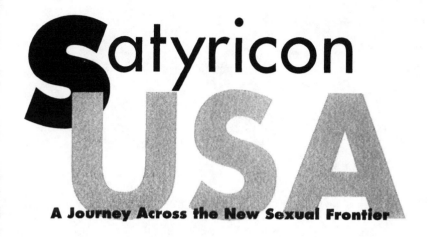

Satyricon USA

A Journey Across the New Sexual Frontier

Eurydice

A Touchstone Book
Published by Simon & Schuster
New York London
Sydney Singapore

TOUCHSTONE
Rockefeller Center
1230 Avenue of the Americas
New York, NY 10020

The Library of Congress has cataloged the Scribner edition
as follows:
Eurydice.
Satyricon: a journey across the new sexual
frontier/Eurydice.
p.   cm.
1. Sex—United States—Philosophy.
2. Sex customs—United States.
3. Sex—Moral and ethical aspects—United States.
4. United States—Social conditions.
I. Title.
HQ18.U5E83   1999
306.7'0973—dc21   98-46448
CIP

ISBN 0-684-83951-2
0-684-86249-2 (Pbk)

Deep, tender thanks to Randall for so much,
to my parents for everything,
to the friends who guided me through
obscure communities or drafts,
and to Heather Schroder, Biz Mitchell, and
Bob Guccione Jr. for first imagining this

Contents

Introduction: Sex Across America   *11*

Provincetown: Guys as Dolls   *21*

New York: Masters of Ceremony   *44*

Pensacola: War in Peace   *67*

San Francisco: Blood Simple Babes   *90*

Dallas: The Economy of Desire   *115*

Cincinnati: Intercourse by Numbers   *135*

Americans Abroad: Virgins at Heart   *157*

Los Angeles: Tales from the Crypt   *181*

Miami and Santa Fe: Alien Romance   *197*

Memphis: Hypercoitus   *218*

A Postscript   *246*

Notes   *251*

"We have complicated every simple gift of the gods."
                                        Diogenes, c. 456 B.C.

Introduction:
Sex Across America

As the first century of Christianity was coming to a close, Titus Petronius Arbiter, governor of Bithynia, purveyor of taste at Nero's notorious parties, and "a scientist of pleasure," was accused of conspiracy. Knowing the range of Nero's rage, Petronius severed his veins and then bandaged them to relish his death; he dined, joked with friends, recited frivolous poems, made a list of the emperor's debaucheries, which he sealed for posterity, and dozed off, so his death would look natural. Legend has it that, before he fell asleep, he wrote, sitting in his bathtub, the entire *Satyricon*. Out of its 2,000 pages, some 250 survive in fragments.

Petronius liked the chaos of human sexuality and blamed the Greco-Roman separation of mind and body, which our culture has inherited, for the persecutions of his protagonist Encolpius (Crotch) by the vengeful god of lust. The *Satyricon* is a satyr's odyssey, with the hero suffering the wrath of the god Priapus in brief erotic episodes. The book is also a subtle denunciation of a Rome turned narcissistic through the loss of its Republican values to the lure of Mammon. The writer depicts an everyday reality of pimps, bureaucrats, pederasts, soldiers, courtesans, slaves; a multicultural world where moneylenders talk in poetry, whores are powerful priests, boyfriends and wives are constantly abducted, corpses get eaten, and professors dress in drag: in short, "a landscape infested with divinity." "It is simple realism and nothing more," Petronius wrote in his own defense.

The extant *Satyricon* opens with Encolpius complaining that schools shield us from reality. Ignoring his professor's retort, he runs away from college, but he can't find his own house anymore, and this confusion is the outset of his orgiastic adventures. To my surprise, this was pretty much my own experience with this book. Having been in universities since the age of fifteen, I left them in 1995 to write it—driven by a desire to both compensate for the sensational sleazy confessions that had become the norm of our sexual discourse and to understand the sources of our fascination. My research took me on an extraordinary rite-of-passage road trip through America. I saw a home I didn't quite recognize. In school I had learned and taught that America was becoming frightfully neoconservative, and then that America was becoming reassuringly politically correct; I found neither to be accurate. What I encountered were mostly ancient, confining sexual mores going by new, emancipatory names. So that became my subject: the tricky disguise of our self-denials as sexual excesses.

> *"What we cannot speak about, we must pass over in silence."*
>
> *Ludwig Wittgenstein,* Tractatus

"My most memorable sexual experience," I told a congregation of upper-middle-class wives in Providence, Rhode Island, one cold weekend afternoon, "was during Easter in Crete." These women ran a social group dedicated to unshackling their sexualities by "mutual sacred exploration." I'd been

12

invited by the 230-pound wife of a surgeon, mother of school-children, and interior decorator. We'd begun by evoking Isis, Aphrodite, Cybele, dipping our fingers in bowls of oil, casting from our bodies impure fears, and holding hands and squatting round a candle-festooned table. As a warm-up to their bonding sexploration, they went round the circle evoking positive sexual experiences to draw strength and inspiration. "To tell our stories is to come out of isolation and honor pleasure as a gift from God," the hostess urged. The attention of the listeners, the fuming incense, and the joint confirmation that followed every telling made the tales more weighty than they were.

"I was visiting a friend whose house overlooked a church," I said in my turn. "As crowds gathered in the pavilion and priests in golden robes sang Byzantine psalms and passed the holy flame, we two stood on the balcony over the congregation and he kissed me. It was a surprise. By the time the priests sang the resurrection hymn, 'Christ has risen from the dead, stepping on the death of death, giving eternal life,' his arms were around my hips, and my body leaned off the balcony. The crowds were kissing, cheering, shooting fireworks; the bells of every church were ringing. I felt that I had risen from the dead, I was stepping on a little death of death, and I was eternal."

The women sat still; they had been raised in families where sex was equated with sin, but they also felt a reverence for sex as a source of life. Then the hostess beamed and said this was what the group strove for: to return meaning to sex without being trapped in tyrannical clichés. The decorator, resplendent in her white reclining nudity, declared that this was everyone's sexual agenda at the end of our millennium: to make sex sacred and thus morally free. "For me, sex is a manifestation of spiritual need," I assented. "I can't actually explain it." And that is my theory of sexuality.

After chanting an ode, the hostess extolled us to "reconnect with our neglected bodies, renounce memories of fear or shame, and assist each other's sexual journey, knowing that the soul's hunger for ecstasy is as real and urgent as the body's hunger for pleasure." The complexity of the emotions pulsating about the dim room, the haphazard crisscrossing of wants and wills, oppressed me. This was the world I'd undertaken to record. Some women wept as if in the bowels of despair. Others held them. Then their soothing touches turned fingertip-light and sneakily erotic, their faces hard and determined. Some convulsed, some danced lewdly, some rolled on the floor, kicking and laughing. It occurred to me that two hundred years ago every woman here would have been burned. And yet I had the eerie sense that ritual was another protective device used to circumscribe our sexual conduct and save us from disappearing into each other, as if what we fell in love with were imaginary black holes.

It was early 1996. America's sexuality felt liminal and exuberant. Fertility drugs, sperm banks, in vitro walk-ins, had divorced sex from procreation. Coital pleasure was seen as an end in itself. More people demanded gratification. Gays, lesbians, and transsexuals were "coming out," exposing families and colleagues to multiform sexualities. Young people fetishized lived-in, pierced, tattooed flesh. Older people drove across country on cyberdates. New Agers practiced tantric yoga. The fear of death-by-sex had subsided and, in typical millennial style, death-and-sex had become a form of recreational kink. Movies glamorized hot-wax sex, car-crash sex. Porn videos were swapped in school buses and watched at slumber parties. Academia was plundering sexual testimonies for topics, and scholars were denouncing the veiled body as analogous to covert government actions and were conferencing on S/M. The feminist shibboleths that the personal is political and secrecy is oppression had touched America's individualist nerve. Old sexual contracts were breaking down, rendering our neatest fixed preconceptions obsolete. The next phase of the sexual revolution was expected to shift the homo-hetero dichotomy toward an inclusive polysexuality. It seemed conceivable that in our lifetime Catholic priests would marry, housewives would swap dildos like recipes, and sex would be seen as a celebration of life rather than a harbinger of trauma, disease, etc.

At the same time, a new type of sexual repression had surreptitiously emerged. A six-year-old boy in Lexington, North Carolina, and a seven-year-old in Brooklyn, New York, were suspended for sexual harassment after kissing female schoolmates on the cheek. Eighty-one percent of polled eighth to eleventh graders felt they had been sexually harassed. Antioch College in Ohio published a code of sexual conduct for students that required verbal consent at every stage of intimacy. Army recruits, corporate suits, and Mitsubishi factory workers in Normal, Illinois, were made to attend sexual ethics seminars. New Haven masons were warned to abide by a "five-second rule": if they looked at a female colleague for more than five seconds, it could be sexual harassment. An executive was fired for recounting a "Seinfeld" episode to a female colleague. A Nebraska graduate student was forced to remove from his desk a photo of his wife in a bikini. The U.S. Supreme Court allowed an Arkansas woman to take the president of the United States to court on uncorroborated charges of sexual harassment; as she had not been fired, demoted, or deprived of benefits, her real charge was impropriety. Having shed the stranglehold of sin, America was devising more sexual rules than were prescribed at any time in this century. These ever-broader definitions of rape signaled a compulsion for regulation that followed each moral laxity we achieved. Caught in the old struggle between the need to satisfy our desires and the need to test our souls, or between the needs of society and of the species, we set ourselves strictest principles of conduct—for we still understood sex as transgression. Our mushrooming draconian guidelines were redefining the private desires of citizens as issues of public legal control, marking the reincarnation of America's inherited puritanism in a more modern, tolerable garb, and solidifying our desires into traps.

For some time, I had considered our current restrictions to be the expected extreme vacillations of a culture in the process of finding a less coherent and more tolerant moral balance. We still had no philosophy, theology, pedagogy, or literature of sexuality. Our public morality was an incoherent collection of contradictory archaic views bequeathed to us from eras otherwise forgotten. We were inventing a new ethos, and were bound to falter and exaggerate until we became carnally literate. But I now had to admit that our outspokenness was not a victory for oppressed sexualities, and didn't promote a proliferation of sexual options; it was a frustrating struggle to conquer, even deny, nature. Our candid articulation had become a repository of tropes and dictums that justified repression, and our vast sexual discourse only reinforced our awareness of sex as danger. I worried our new byzantine structures bent the scales too much on the sectarian side of fairness and reason. I feared the emptiness at the heart of our sexual demystification. As sex became associated with gender war, paranoia, a panacea, or a thesis for our general being, the simple joys of tactile, olfactory, visual, and aural immersion in one another were becoming skewed or neglected.

It was the time when a Brown University student was expelled on an unfounded charge of sexual harassment, and most polled undergraduates agreed that a mere charge should suffice to incur punishment. As I walked by that venerable university citadel, I felt that, by taking no stance, I was implicated in a witch-hunt. I decided our new openness was dividing rather than unifying us, pitting our grievances against one another rather than against the system that bore them.

"You think we don't know about sex out here, but we know all there is," a Mennonite elder told me a few months later in Sugarcreek, Ohio. "We don't discuss it because we have no need to. We all know what to do." The land was rolling gold-green and fertile and his as far as the eye could see. We were rocking in wooden chairs, digesting a lavish lunch. He said he saw no need for anyone to interfere with what people did in private. I asked his granddaughter, a young nurse who mostly stared at the vast sky, if she knew all she needed to about sex. "My girlfriends and I . . . we know all about it. We don't do it, because we don't want to be taken advantage of. Having my own voice is more important to me than having sex. My boyfriend understands." "She's a feminist," Grampa grumbled. Her modern logic kept her as chaste as her faith would once have.

> "It takes a mind debauched by learning to carry the process of making the natural seem strange so far as to ask for the 'why' of any instinctive act."
> William James, The Varieties of Religious Experience

When I began my research, I was intrigued by America's growing sexual fringe. What interested me was the prospect, inherent in every society, that in time the social margins would expand enough to become the status quo. I interviewed many paraphiliacs,* looking for the source of their commitment to nonmainstream pleasure. I soon realized I had exaggerated their differences. Most struck me as the Masons or Dungeons & Dragons buffs of previous generations. What they did in private might qualify as morally flawed or abnormal, but they did not.† For some, sexual aberration was like a cruise: an adventure. For many, deviation provided a means of sculpting a self out of a homogenized world, so they embraced it vehemently. For most, sexual eccentricity was just a way to be and feel interesting. For all their talk about overcoming outdated limits and the "tyranny of the majority," they were looking to escape

---

*Paraphilia is a tendency or an appetite for atypical forms of sexual intimacy. Webster's Third International Dictionary defines it as "an addiction to peculiar or bizarre sexual practice."
†Throughout this book, I use normal as a statistical term.

the drab frustrations of ordinary civilized life, and sex is the one foolproof way humanity has had to feel whole, incandescent, and alive.

I met transvestites who every dawn serviced Hassidim merchants on their way to work because their faith forbade sex with women but not ex-men; I met sex-addicted priests, and Christian virgins who were anally promiscuous; I met teens who studied mortuary science because they had come to realize, after an average heartbreaking love life, that the dead held more romantic allure than the living; I met models who believed abstinence made them look sexier, businesswomen who served their menstrual blood in meatloaf dishes at dinner parties to snag mates, lesbians who bled themselves in orgasm, nymphomaniacs who struggled with sexual aversion; I met lawyers who paid to be electroshocked during their lunch hour, bankers who dressed as cheerleaders during their lunch hour, politicians who liked to be hung on a cross, bagpipers (armpit-sex), genuphallators (knee-sex), furtlers (sex with pictures of celebrities), pygmalionists (sex with mannequins); I attended workshops where burly truckers learned to perform "sacred spot massage," and sexuality camps where yuppie couples studied felching. And in the end, the S/M dungeons I visited were no more libidinally intense and no less hospitable than the bare-walled homes of Amish bishops.

I saw that, up close, the outrageousness of the most unacceptable sexual practice vanishes into the ordinariness of the human being who engages in it. So whenever I found myself in a state of uncertainty and apprehension, I went by the assumption that, as Plato says in the *Symposium*, "where there is mutual consent, there is what the law proclaims to be right." And the less I questioned, the more I was told, and the less I judged, the more I was trusted. The great undersung virtue of the American society is the openness of its people. Strangers confided in me generously, with no guarantee of being favorably presented, out of a genuine desire for commemoration.

And despite their serendipitous congruencies, these people couldn't be reduced to systems of reactions or fetishes or aesthetics. The plethora of their private needs taught me that sexuality can be neither delimited nor defined.

My personal attitude today is that sex should be neither underestimated nor overinterpreted, neither shamefully hidden nor publicly broadcast. My favorite definition of sex is William James's definition of religious experience: "The mystical feeling of enlargement, union, and emancipation [that] has no specific intellectual content of its own . . . the abandonment of self-responsibility." Only a dreary mind can't leave mystery alone.

My primary project here is not to depict problematic contemporary sexual practices, trace their evolution, and analyze the ideas that drive them; it is to present a record of a long, tentative study, at the end of which I came to think and perceive intimacy differently from the way I had before. My main topic is America. I'm interested in what we don't talk about when we talk about sex—starting with the panhistoric assumption that sexual desire is the beast lurking in our social jungle whose containment is the prerequisite for a moral, stable civilization; and ending with the suggestion that sex is used in our public life as a loud distraction from important practical, emotional, and ideological issues. Because this is not a scholarly book, I have not weighed it down with references to the books and articles that were my invaluable sources. I tape-recorded (openly and with permission) the interviews and naturally occurring discourse in all but the most sensitive cases. What appears in quotes or paraphrase also exists on tape or notepad. I abridged and edited quotes, condensed time and sequence, consolidated locations and characters, rearranged names, ages, and occupations to protect my sources' valued anonymity, and to compose comprehensive archetypes representative of the people I met in each "scene." I certainly do not presume to understand any individuals. At best, this book aspires to capture our psychic anatomy in a textual snapshot of our moment in history and to illustrate part of the sexual nerve pulsing across America. I expect that all I can say will fall short of the subject. The rest is realism, and nothing more.

Provincetown: Guys as Dolls

"J'est un autre."*
    Arthur Rimbaud, in a letter to Georges Izambard, 1871

At a writers' conference auspiciously titled "Unspeakable Practices," I met the writer Toby Olsen when I was mistakenly assigned to his Victorian bed-and-breakfast room; making small talk, I mentioned an offer I'd just received to write a book about American sexuality. I told him I couldn't imagine a voice and style that would "be true to" sex and also refreshing and useful. Toby warmed to the subject, gleefully describing the transformation of his fishing town every October when "she-men" took it over. He offered me the use of his house, phone numbers, and clips, and I felt he would be disappointed if I didn't write about it, so I called the organizers to inquire. A prohibitively serious man introduced himself as a woman on the phone and advised me to read up on the subject, and soon enough a dozen books with titles like Fantasies Can Set You Free arrived in the mail. I decided I might as well pack.

I like asking questions. I like quantities of people and stories. I always want to know what they do, where they come from, how

*"I is an other."

they like themselves, what meaning they ascribe to life. And people of all kinds, including the most disturbing, always talk to me. This was why I thought I might be able to write this book.

The "she-men" I met cheerfully mothered me and fawned over my intrusive inquisitiveness. Given a guarantee of anonymity, they rushed to confess, seeing no courage in silence. It was as if to hold their tongues would be to license a great wrong. Unedited salacious information poured my way. This was possibly America's most useful and most destructive tenet: the confidence or conceit that everything can be understood.

A Novice's Glossary

FI (female impersonator); TV (transvestite); CG (cross-gender); TS (transsexual); AN (androgyne); BIG (bigenderist); SRS (sex reassignment surgery); FTM (surgically reassigned female-to-male); MTF (surgically reassigned male-to-female); CGC (conscious-gender community). Cross-dressers prefer to be addressed in the feminine pronoun. (I overlook this rule in good conscience, in order to depict more accurately my reactions to these people.)

The ballroom stage rattles under three gargantuan figures in flowing sequined dresses, butterfly eyelashes, and cascading hairpieces, striking poses to "Dancing Queen." They smile, mingling coquetry with secret alert, and shimmy flamboyantly. The audience, shoulder-to-shoulder thick, cheers as the performers (nicknamed the Andrews Sisters) are followed by a Divine lookalike in rhinestone mumu lip-synching "Hawaiian Hula." On the floor, the reigning aesthetic is Barbara Bush polyester-and-pearls. The revelers are tax attorneys, cardiologists, building contractors, nuclear engineers, computer programmers, network executives, library presidents, in thousands of dollars' worth of womanly gear, united by their blind faith in the power of appearances. A mass of disparate sculptured parts and ironic cultural fragments, they are joined in a pandemic erotic discontent, a yearning to be lifted out of their ordinary lives, a fondly premeditated masculine rebellion.

Fantasia Fair, held every October in Provincetown, Massachusetts, offers eighty seminars and "talent and fashion shows" during a week of cross-dressing in public. This year it is attended by 120 mostly middle-aged heterosexual men who stand to lose a lot of social power if they are discovered. They come to this out-of-the-way town to find relief from the requirements of workaholic masculinity and feel fortified in their numbers. Their "femme-persona" lets them forget their banes and body aches and chills of mortal reckoning. They are like *Tootsie*-clad Promise Keepers: a semireligious gathering of men weary of their inability to touch and be touched, looking for unconditional fraternity, respect, love.

Phyllis breaks the snaking conga line on the floor to give me a welcoming hug. "I'd love to share my bed with you," she says jovially, taking me aside. "We have eighteen millionaires here," she explains confidentially. "They've done all they wanted to do in life. Now they want the best of both worlds. That's what we help them with. Since 1973, we have been teaching people boundaries are only in our minds. We take our role-modeling very seriously."

The fair is organized by support groups like the International Foundation for Gender Education (IFGE), Transgenderists Independence Club (TGIC), Tiffany Club, Outreach Institute for Gender Studies, Transgender Nation, Monmouth Ocean Transgender, FTM International, and Society for the Second Self (Tri-Ess). The fair's headquarters are in the windswept, daintily restored Pilgrim House hotel in this fishing village–cum–summer resort of three thousand, where the Puritans first landed and held to a starving bivouac for months before proceeding to Plymouth Rock, not suspecting their descendants would one day interpret the meaning of "the free and the brave" to include gender-rearranging. Yet, like the

Puritans, cross-dressers do what they believe they have to do, regardless of personal sacrifice. They, too, are loners who follow strident inner voices. They, too, have mostly meek wives persevering on the sidelines and pompous charismatic leaders; they, too, presume the body can be tamed; and they, too, believe they are building the better society of the future.

As many as 15 million heterosexual American men are cross-dressers. Conservative estimates place them at 3 to 5 percent of the male population. From corporate presidents to athletes, they represent the range of American society; they live in suburbs and barrios, teach Sunday school and lead Boy Scouts. Most research suggests the behavior is determined by parental identification patterns. A study in the *Journal of the American Psychoanalytic Association* links cross-dressing to a need to disassociate from pressures of masculinity via fantasy, a symptom called "lesbian preoccupation" (once called the Oedipus complex). Other studies point to a genetic predisposition or an in utero hormonal imbalance; the Y-hypothesis contends the cross-dresser's embryo has less Y chromosome pushing the gonads to become testes; the prenatal symbiotic fusion theory proposes the cross-dresser subconsciously holds memories of the warm womb life that it relives "enfemme." The cross-dressers themselves also bring up anything from cutting-edge neurological brain research ("a guerrilla segment of the cerebellum") to the genome project ("the cross-dressing gene") to B. F. Skinner ("It's all determined," they assure me, "by the age of three").

Tonight the ballroom door is manned by a smiling boy who only a year ago was a butch in paste-on whiskers. She took hormones to sprout a wispy beard and had breast reduction and a penis constructed from her wrist bone. "All of it can be reversed," he says happily. This neo-Tiresias and his partner have been monogamous for eight years. They started off as a lesbian couple, became a heterosexual one after his partner's gender reassignment, and are now a gay pair. The past is inconsequential, the slate perennially clean: it is the embodiment of postmodernity.

Melanie is a thirty-eight-year-old university professor in Durham, North Carolina, a leading paleontologist and father of four teenage girls. Erica is a forty-four-year-old marketer for DuPont in Wilmington, Delaware. Paula is a forty-year-old Seattleite, a digital trendologist, Lutheran ex-missionary, father of three children. All are normal enough to have first found out about other cross-dressers in an article in *Playboy* (Paula), a *Penthouse* letter (Erica), and an Ann Landers column. All three talk in a composed nasal drone that I learn is a "femme" voice. We're having midnight dinner at the Flagship restaurant after the "Follies" amateur revue.

"People, even cross-dressers, fear the chaos of androgyny," Melanie is saying. "Our leaders run the fair like a stuffy sorority with uplifting talks and refreshments. But cross-dressing is *sexual*." Melanie's wife doesn't support his dressing so he's getting a divorce; he doesn't plan to "come out" to anyone else, but he dreams of meeting a bisexual woman willing to fist him. I ask him to explain the sexuality of cross-dressing. "My therapist says I resent women for having the power to attract me sexually by looking a certain way; by appropriating their tools, I take back my power." Is sex a power struggle between desired and desirer? And are women in control by being the ones who get objectified, paraded, penetrated? "At the macro level, the phallus rules," he admits. "But in domestic life, women rule. My mother and sister were beautiful. I wore their clothes until my dad beat me and hammered into me how wrong it was. We learn early that beauty is power, beauty is feminine, so 'sex' is feminine. Male is boring, reductionist, utilitarian. Men are mules. It's why I can't understand gay men. When men are attracted to me as a woman, I feel no desire. I'm attracted to *myself* as a woman. My sexuality is in self-absorption. When a Hollywood star enters a room, everyone is at her feet. That's the power I want and can't have as a man. If someone tells me 'You're absolutely ravishing,' I get an erection. I feel desirable as a woman because my male attractiveness is alien to me as a guy. But women find me attractive as a man. So those who desire me I don't desire and those I desire don't desire me as I want to be desired." Is this his tragedy? "Yes. I spent twenty-five years depressed. I held every school record in track and field. I worked as a ski instructor in Utah, where I wasn't tempted by women's clothes and ads. Then my dad died. I dressed right after the funeral and had a professional makeup. Now, I'm Cinderella; I go to the ball, then rub the ash back on."

Paula agrees: "Men are hairy, bulky, dirty. I wouldn't want to have sex with one. I grew up in redneck Oklahoma. I put on my mom's skirt and masturbated. I had to hold off so I wouldn't spill on her clothes. In college I married a Mormon. It took me ten years to dare put on my wife's lipstick and masturbate. Now she gets horny when she makes me up. We have a great sex life. *I* wear her panties." He crinkles his foxy face. He has his own permed hair, monkstrap shoes, a plain pleated dress. "I go to Sunday mass as Paula," he boasts. "I dress around my sons. My oldest went to a costume party as a girl. My brothers all cross-dressed as kids—birdseed for breasts, rope for wigs, food coloring, the works."

It doesn't take long to realize cross-dressers are good citizens: they are hard workers, ardent consumers, have model jobs, strong families, money in the bank—all the trophies of normalcy and formidable willpower. Cross-dressing doesn't threaten the operations of society, even though it depends on duplicity. Unlike drag queens, who are sexually drawn to men and emulate bombshells, cross-dressers are sexually attracted to women and emulate females who surrender their libidos to social proprieties. Theirs is a straight man's idea of womanhood: love to tease, hate to put out.

"I'm a Buddhist," Erica is saying. "Getting dressed is my

meditation. It's bliss." With red ponytail, ostrich legs, and a gawky body in a plaid librarian's dress, he resembles the celluloid Olive Oyl. "I'm a typical baby boomer, I know the president of MCI, the vice president of MTV. I'm an Orlando. My lesbian girlfriend is proper, controlled, no makeup. My sex life is a fantasy world I make up for myself, tailor-made just for me. My girlfriends have told me my body represents the godhead—the unification of opposites. They tell me sexually I'm a national treasure."

Eric, a Yale man, is descended from George Washington; he played sax in a big band, published poetry, volunteered at Samaritan House, married a known debutante, and handled Kmart's $500 million video distribution account. One year he sold more Disney videos than any other person in the world, which got him a job with Disney in marketing, where a lesbian colleague encouraged his cross-dressing. He longed to shed his male uniform for "Erica's pretty things" and got a divorce, conceding his property to his spouse to avoid having his cross-dressing come out in court. His ex-wife remarried, then sued Eric for molesting his son. A search warrant produced a dildo, and photos of Erica. "They had no proof outside the credibility of an imaginative five-year-old who liked Disney movies and was treated as an independent objective eyewitness," he says. "We all have dark images in our subconscious. But I had no stomach for a court battle, and the legal system would tear my son to shreds. I took a plea bargain: thirty years probation, eight hundred hours community service, sex offender program—which you complete only if you admit being an offender. And I'm not allowed to see my son until he's of age. He is the person I love most in the world, and I haven't seem him in ten years." I ask if he has regrets about losing his son for Erica. "No, I lost him to discrimination. Drag is a way to gain power, a defense. I'm shy, but in drag I'm a vicious queen bitch, I feel untouchable. What I've learned by going out as a female helps me as a male—I'm more self-reliant now." In a perverse way, cross-dressing is an affirmation of masculinity: in his camouflage, Eric infiltrates "femininity" to reinforce his manhood.

"Melanie," says Melanie, "has no responsibilities, no kids, no parents; she can handle more liquor than Mel, smokes, laughs loud. I get to live two lives; I eat of the tree of knowledge."

The first Fantasia workshop I attend is a political update, and I am the only "genetic girl" in the room. This morning the audience reminds me of Hassidim wives: long skirts, wigs, scarves, gold earrings, big glasses, a heaviness of bearing. They sit with hands clasped demurely on their laps, chins up, respectable, placid, keen, brittle, and purposefully messianic—like unerotic mother figures.

Virginia Prince sits stiffly in the front row wearing red ribbons in her platinum tresses and red earrings, red mini, and red blouse that reveals a lacy bra underneath. Her eyes are steely and unforgiving, and clash disconcertingly with her expert wrist twists and attention-getting mannerisms. Her lipstick is smeared over Popeyeishly snarled lips, in the habit of old ladies. She seems half senile girlhood, half impertinent virility. At eighty-five, she is the hero of this group. After living as a man for fifty-five years and divorcing twice, he went on hormones in 1967 and sold his chemist's business to live as a woman, "in order to complete [his] perception of human life." She started the first social group for CDs, the Tiffany Club, in 1977, and the first major CD magazine and press in 1981.

"Gender is an anachronism," the guest speaker is saying. In the nature versus nurture debate, CDs are firmly pro-nurture; they know that *being* a woman doesn't guarantee possession of the idealized "feminine" powers they covet. "The gender line is the prejudice our society values most, for the sake of family. But sex is between the legs, gender between the ears. Anatomy is the last frontier. The body *will* change in the twenty-first century." It is a unifying motif of our age: the confidence that technology, mimicking the complex ebb and flow of nature, will hijack evolution; as the A, C, G, and T of DNA join the digital 0 and 1, the boundary between the given and the made will be blissfully extinguished.

The attentive men gathered here have a political platform. They want Congress to endorse an "International Bill of Gender Rights" affirming people's right to choose their gender and still marry and raise children; they want formal education to recognize "the trans struggle," toilets not to be marked by gender, sex categories to be removed from identification papers. They believe the "two-party sexual system is in defiance of nature." "Gender liberation" is their heroic cause. "We have faced what frightens so many: our inner femininity," Virginia says. "We've met this erstwhile enemy and made a degree of peace with her. Androgyny is an act of resistance."

"I saw it all in the fifties and sixties," Phyllis tells me in the tone of a burned-out veteran. "The police raided bars and arrested cross-dressers on felony charges until 1969." That turning point was the famous Stonewall Rebellion, a four-night drag queen uprising in Greenwich Village that brought attention to the senseless criminalization of transvestites. "In the sixties my friend Euphrosyne had an apartment in New York with two doors: he'd enter in his pilot's uniform and leave as a woman. A drag queen called the cops on him. They arrested him under an arcane law that was designed to forbid Indians from going in public with face paint. He lost the case, appealed four times, and lost each time until 1973, when the law was repealed. In 1973 they didn't let queens in the Gay Day parade. Today the gays don't let CDs in. We get bashed by gays. We're where the gays were in 1970."

Now the audience is discussing "reverse sexism." "Women have worn crew cuts for years," Erica argues. "If a woman puts on slacks, it's OK. If a man puts on a dress, he has gender issues." "*We* fulfill our procreational duties," Paula says. "We should be allowed more freedom than gays, not less." "Lesbians should be on our side," Erica insists. "They shun us in disregard of sisterly community. Women are now the establishment. We want equality. We want to be able to do what women do, not *be* women." "The women's movement started all this," Phyllis tells me. "When women came out in the corporate world dressed like men, men took cross-dressing seriously."

The discussion ends abruptly when a man in a skewed bob and ill-fitting housedress takes the floor. "I have White House credentials," he brags, holding hands with a weathered wife who stands by him in Army fatigues, "CIA clearance, Secret Service experience, I'm a Rotarian, a Mason, an ex-Marine. No one here knows my name. If my neighbors saw me, they wouldn't know me. My feet are swollen; my earlobes hurt; my back aches; I don't spend as much time as I should on my makeup. But I'm grateful to be one of you. You're respectable taxpayers. *We* run this country." He's not adept enough to modify his gruff soldiery voice, and people roll their eyes snobbishly. He's Archie Bunker in blue eyeshadow. I think of the dresses in J. Edgar Hoover's closet.

On their way out, the participants stop and brazenly study me. What are they looking for? "A woman is a composite," Phyllis tells me in the congenial manner of a connoisseur of robots at an expo. "*We* haven't gone through girlhood, menstruation, childbirth, the labia folds, the G-spot stuff. All that is built into your femininity, the way you comport yourself. Look at the way you're sitting: a wonderful casual pose. Women smile more—a gesture of submission—and move their lips and keep their fingers unevenly spaced." This makes me feel leaden, ineptly unaware of the puppet chains of my predetermined animation. I feel I am artificial, like a chemistry equation.

Afterward, Phyllis regally ushers me to her room, a combination ransacked guerrilla headquarters and aging lady's rancid boudoir. In sunlit close-up, her face is all cracked lips and heavy flaring brows, drained cheekbones and rough skin. Aged laugh lines hinge her chin. Every so often, to show her malaise at the perils and entanglements of life, her eyes shut and the pink tip of her tongue slides out tiredly and her face encompasses the hopelessness of all human knowing. But her nails stay impeccably glossy, red, and hard, her fingers keep pointing, her head shakes on involuntarily. Her eyes glimmer predatorily as she proposes that I should write her biography.

"I gave up astrophysics and became a professional gender counselor because I *love* my sisters for allowing their feminine feelings out," she explains after the obligatory briefing on her life story. "We're more human than most men; we're a generation ahead of society. Now I advise the neophytes. I have a protégée who sends out strong sexual signals as a feminine and sisters want to relate to her sexually, maybe do sixty-nine with the penises; I discourage that sort of thing. A sister who has sex with another can't take the guilt and looks for release in drink or drugs. Males don't know their sexuality. Cross-dressers are so afraid of homosexuality they prefer to look in the mirror and feel 'I'm the most beautiful princess in the universe' and leave it at that; they don't even know how to touch themselves outside the penis. Sisters are naive about the diversity of sex. So when their adrenaline kicks in, and endorphins mix in, it can be explosive—especially when a mental sign says 'Red light! Are you homosexual? Plus, AIDS. Plus, what will I tell my wife?' " If they can tell their wives they cross-dress, I assume the rest is easy. "Wives are what parents were: moral poles. Emotionally, sisters are preteens. If you dress like a twelve-year-old girl, chances are you feel like one. We get crushes, we get scared, don't know how to respond, and worry about the day after. As a woman, I don't want a one-night stand. I'm giving my body up with great respect for it and for you. I'll only let you explore parts of me that are private because I feel you'll honor that with dignity." Judging from his lip licking and lowered suggestive timbre, I think he is seducing me as a mother superior would a young parishioner, in a roundabout, spider-and-fly way. When I meet his gaze, he assumes an absentminded expression, lids down to emphasize the lined lashes and hide his predatory signs. I suspect matronly women's clothes give him an excuse to be lascivious in a politically correct way.

"This culture thinks a push-pull-click is sex. It's bestial. It's not l-o-v-e. And I love to see your glistening eyes taking me in." And I recognize this unrealistic voice addressing me: patriarchy, sustained on the chimeras of male chivalry, female modesty, the honor of virginity, the inevitability of true love. Like a conservative Christian, Phyllis defines the female body as a social treasure that must be sealed off, safeguarded, rationed carefully and stingily; it's the old concern that if women give away the milk for free, men won't bother to buy the cow, the fear that has kept women faithful, inexperienced, selfless.

Inside her narrow bathroom, Phyllis retouches her makeup as she talks, and I play the part of an awed ten-year-old watching the mysterious, confidential ritual of the private concoction of grown-up femininity. She runs to and from her brimming closet in her underwear and rummages for outfits (it's the custom of the fair to change clothes a few times a day), acting out the intimacy between two airheaded ingenues getting ready for a ball. Our roles keep switching too quickly for me to keep up. He towers over me and helplessly asks me to zip his gown, his muscular body amended into an inflexible hourglass by a pointy padded bra and padded girdles. "This is a caftan my spouse sewed for me in 1976. She was a pioneer in gender. I chose my wife because of her wardrobe. I worried how she would take my fixation, but she got so involved with it, I let her have a ball. She shops for it, it's a fun project for her, like redecorating; I am her life-sized Barbie. A compliment to my looks is a tribute to her work. This cape I wore on a panel when Leonard Bernstein hit on me and I felt real vulnerable; I spurned him." He puts on a black lace bra over his prostheses, a rubbery belt, a second pair of latex panties, Q-size panty-hose, looking increasingly like an NFL lineman. "It is like being in a straitjacket. Oh, get me out! But, if I like a little more hip, I can add more hip," he explains merrily.

He takes visible pleasure in being "naked" around me, showing off his metamorphosis. But our chat isn't really that of two women getting ready to go out; we're more like a father and son at work on the family car: "While we wait for these things to dry," he says of his freshly repainted nails, "I need you to hand me that glue. These babies are what we call prostheses: 38C, 36C, 34B. Props are mental aids. If my penis is tucked away in a jockstrap, I go into no-penis mentality. Sex is about presentation. Real breasts are sickly extraneous ligaments." He makes me touch them. They are soft and strong. "Oh, you hurt me!" he jokes girlishly. "Now let me touch yours." Underneath the layers of talk and pad and paint, a man's gaze is searching me out, objectifying and staking me.

Erica takes me to a wives' support group so I can hear the "genetic angle." Like Phyllis, Erica perennially wears the morose stare of motherly prototypes that says this woman was put on this earth to suffer. All around us, groups of cross-dressers buoyantly and gingerly dash out of shops with packages of trailing muslin scarves and infections of glee, looking battle-stunned. They greet us with profuse assertions of affected camaraderie and fondness. Their idealized sisterhood frightens me because it's a delusional wish for innocence inside a synthetic Eden; it's how I imagine the tyranny of Peter Pan.

We find a dozen prim wives sitting in a circle. "We have no one to talk to about this problem," the mediator is saying, "except each other. My best friends are CD wives. We go on vacations, eat out, together. We know clothes don't make the man. My husband is as lovable in my clothes as in his. He's actually nicer as a femme, more kind, loving, *real.* He's a good father, husband, friend, provider. So it was his lifelong fantasy to find a woman who'd love his femme; I fulfilled it. He'll never forget that. And he's faithful. If he has shaved legs, he won't fool around." I can't see why a man needs makeup to be kind and "real." "Because of society's stereotypes," she answers easily, "our conditioning. It's only fair for him to put on dresses if I wear pants. If I can be a good sheriff *and* wife and mother, he deserves the same latitude." But she doesn't go by a male name as a sheriff, doesn't wear padding to feign a penis, doesn't lower her voice to a baritone, and doesn't get off on it. "I don't have to. I'm free to enter the men's world. For him, *beauty* and *virtue* are forbidden. It's not an easy time to be a man." I agree with that. But does all this baroque "dressing" help us accept the reality of male "femininity"? "I don't love the *visible* femme," she concedes. "When I found out his secret, I'd decided to leave him. What cleared my preconceived ideas was reading and meeting other CDs."

"My husband was macho," a bouncy obese petite interrupts, "hard, unfeeling. He had a horrible temper and physically abused me. One day we saw a cross-dresser on 'Phil Donahue'; he told me he, too, had this other side. He'd tried to resist it, so he was always angry and absent. His therapist gave him *The TV and His Wife* by Virginia Prince; I read it. When I let him dress, he became a homebody. Now our daughter lends him her clothes. She says 'Pamela' is nicer than 'Dad' and she wants to grow up and be like 'her.' Our marriage has transformed. He has a smile on all the time, helps me around the house. I've become less passive. It helps my self-esteem: he says I'm the most important person in his life, and he wants to emulate *me*. Men's lib has given *me* power."

"Mine used to be kind, and now is selfish," Paula's wife says. "He disregards his masculine looks, which is how people see him. He wants to be a femme, but I must clean and pick up after him and change the diapers. When I complain, he switches to Paul and gets bossy. I'd like to be cherished as a woman, too. I can't feel like a woman if he's dressed as a glamour puss every time we make love. Our relationship is what I had with my sister growing up: we shared a room and talked about clothes, makeup, boys. If I didn't have ten years, three kids, the house, the station wagon, I'd bolt."

The youngest wife of the group is even more morose: "I feel cheated, inadequate, rejected—as if my femininity is not enough to satisfy him, he needs his own. I say if he loved me, he'd give this up. He says it's like asking him not to breathe. He says I hold the key to his happiness. I see his pain; I feel mean if I refuse him. I can't win. When I kiss him dressed, I feel guilty. When we have sex, I feel disgust. I married a handsome, strong man and I make love to a fat dyke in burlesque. It's unnatural. All my ideas about marriage have been eroded. That sexy man I'd loved is dead."

"Sexually, we each married a femme," the facilitator confirms. She pronounces everything as if reading a children's story—as if the end of each sentence contained a nice surprise. "Some wives withdraw from sex as a solution. The good news is he trusts you enough to share his secret. Millions of wives are not told. Value his honesty and throw 'normal' out of your vocabulary. A lot worse monsters live in this world. Be glad he's not a drunk, a junkie, a gambler. This is a man's world. If you're not job-trained and have kids, the assets outweigh the liabilities." I realize that, in "feminine" self-abnegation, these wives bow before the needs of their husbands. Men choose, act, achieve; women accept, support, inspire. As always, their security comes at the cost of their sexual happiness.

"I hate the hormones," an older wife says. "I put up with mood swings, tears, nausea, dieting, bulimia. And because of the estrogen, he couldn't orgasm. He didn't care. He said I could have sex with him at will, like my sex doll. I lost it. Then a doctor put him on Caverject. It's a harmless penis shot; it gives him hours of erection. It also comes in a precoital pill. It saved our marriage."

The wives now discuss a luncheon they attended at the home of a local CD's wife who told them cross-dressing is a disease that can be cured by a serotonin pill; she said her feminist psychiatrist considers "dressing" a premeditated game men play on their spouses to "destroy" them. "We must arm against this premeditative ruse against our families," the facilitator urges to quell doubts. "We need strength to protect ourselves. That woman is a snake, spreading discord." In Eden?

According to Greek myth, the sage Tiresias had acquired clairvoyance by divine gender conflict. One day he struck two snakes as they were having sex and became a woman; seven years later he came upon them again, struck them again, and retrieved his former self. Then Zeus and Hera called on him to settle a debate as to whether men or women enjoyed sex more. Tiresias agreed with Zeus that women had greater sexual pleasure, and Hera, in a fit of temper, struck him blind. Zeus, who couldn't undo what another god had done, gave him sight into the future to make up for his loss of sight on earth. In *Oedipus Rex*, Tiresias used it to warn Oedipus of his impending self-blinding. Notably, Oedipus used his mother's brooch to blind himself, after his mother hanged herself by her *scarf*. Freud interpreted Oedipus's self-blinding as an act of self-castration. In a way, cross-dressers are both castrati and visionaries.

Cross-dressers claim various mythic (Ishtar, Hatshepsut, Sardanapalus, Achilles, Hercules) and historical role models: Christine Jorgensen (the GI who had the first publicized sex change in 1952), Chevalier d'Eon (Louis XV's cross-dressing diplomat), Queen Christina of Sweden, Pope Joan/John Anglicus, Saints Marinus (Marina) and Joseph (Hildegund), Joan of Arc, cross-dressing peasant rebels like the Rebeccas in Wales, nineteenth-century female explorers, and Civil War soldiers and guerrillas in male drag. Yet, in previous centuries, "passing" was mostly used by people who needed to escape social inequities and hide their identities. In its current version, "passing" is an expression of identity. It follows in the tradition of seventeenth-century "molly" houses and eighteenth-century drag balls, which were not social rebellions but rather "do as I please" celebrations of the cultural elite.

My impression is that cross-dressers revive the nineteenth-century decorative woman prized for her looks, elegance, demeanor, manners, knowledge of piano-embroidery-French-and–domestic supervision, and her purity. Even if they dress up as Mae West, they want to *be* Clarissa or Jane Eyre. In a world where differences between men and women have begun to dissolve, these men *embody* the women they still long for, ingeniously purloining women back to male possession. Rather than bringing forth a gender-merging synthesis, they retain the confines of binary gender. They bring obsolete femininities, in however parodic a form, back into the culture every time they walk the streets in corsage and corset, impose them on their wives who must compete with their "femmes," pass them to their sons and daughters, expose them to their grandchildren. They keep the stereotypes alive. Their sleight of hand is the vain scaffolding on which they build themselves up as sexually self-sufficient Masters of the Universe.

When I pick her up at her room, Phyllis pulls me inside, appalled. She won't let me go to the Fantasy Ball in the wrinkled black Benetton dress I've worn all day. She advises me to use her curlers ("I put this electric bonnet over my rollers forty-five minutes every morning while I read the paper; I looked for it for years; they don't make them anymore"). She shows me her clothes iron, lotion, toothbrush, shampoo. Sanctimonious and stern, she leaves me to fix myself up. I look through her drawers to confirm that everything there is feminine; it is. I read her *New York Times* until enough time has elapsed to convince her I'm spiffed up, and go down. A crowd at the bottom of the stairs welcomes each new arrival in joyous monosyllables. "What is your fantasy?" they ask everyone.

They fuss over me perplexed until I feel like a disappointing bride. I've come "naked" to a temple of dress. I don't embody a fantasy. I'm naturally padded, at ease in my dress. Isn't that enough?

Inside the ballroom, a twittering harem-girl who is an octogenarian orchid collector waltzes me. "I'm unisex," he prattles. "I go to women's rest rooms but don't have to wait in line at the opera." At the end his crotchety wife bends to put dollar bills in his thigh garter. A "Pocahontas" asks me, "Are you with anyone? Do you have a spouse or are you available?" He gives me his room number ("Come, we'll solve the world's affairs"). "A seventy-year-old can raise a hard-on, but not always ejaculate," he confides. "So, at my age, sex becomes a spiritual quest." He was once a U.S. ambassador in Europe. He now keeps a diary with photos of himself dressed, flyers from conventions, notes from sisters, lists of what he saw, heard, or did "en femme," like any vacationing senior.

"Pamela, your lipstick is smeared," a panicky voice calls out. Pamela writes for the *Philadelphia Inquirer.* He wears a gold lamé number and a wig perched inches above his hairline. His obese wife, in a modest flowery dress, reaches up proprietarily and wipes off his excess lipstick. Wives are a CD's dead giveaway: normally, they are the pliant, sweet women who stand protectively in front of big asexual nondescript guys who look afraid of being hit on by other men. Now the wives lurk in the vicinity, robbed of even their power to be sexual objects, useful only as tutors and accessible resources for mimesis.

The band plays "If You Were a Woman." I dance with Phyllis, who breathes hotly on my nape. Her body feels unhinged, like a mollusk's. She insists that I "lead" our tango, puts my hand on a padded hip, my other hand on a hefty shoulder, and teaches me to push her padding forward and back to make her move to my will. The next song is "Money" by ABBA and we proceed to boogie. I notice she imitates all my moves disorientingly. She also kicks up her thighs, bats her lashes, licks her lips, pats her hair. I am facing a blunt mating prance. "Are you a lesbian?" she asks. It's what everyone here is asking. CDs have much logic invested in my being a woman who desires females. She adds the patronizing cliché, "Did you have a bad experience with a man?" implying a CD could show me better. Yet her dance also strikes me as a *contrapposto* of death. "We're born alone and we die alone," she says in the end. "Drag trains us to be alone." When she walks off, I notice she is bowlegged, like a soccer player.

As bodies sweat away and creatures twirl me about and lift me up, I experience isolated moments of androgynous arousal: I'm attracted by a gauzy black sleeve pulled snug over a broad eagle-tattooed bicep, by hip and thigh muscles flexing unconsciously beneath flimsy white hose, by this singular atmosphere of campiness, animality, *and* decorum. I realize it *could* be exciting if men wore silks and slits to emphasize the attractions of virility. What else is Hercules or Tarzan or Fabio? But as soon as I look at these men with the keenness of desire, their parts disintegrate before my eyes until I'm left with the silly caricatures of a boldface sex object that only a drunk man could covet. I realize their lust is solitary: they only want to be wanted in order to confirm that it's legitimate to want themselves. What they want is to be their own object of desire *and* their own voyeuristic beholder, to be self *and* other, self-contained and coldly complete.

The final night's awards ceremony is by invitation only, but the ex-ambassador lets me in and introduces me around as "the de Tocqueville of gender." He is giggly and plump, with a battered face, fallen jowls, blond teased hair, tweezed arching brows, a fastidious mouth, and the shrewd eyes of a trickster: Al D'Amato in drag. His cleavage is dove-white, baby-soft, lush. "The cross-dresser club I belong to has a budget of half a million; we have a press, bookstore, library; we keep track of every article written on transgenderism," he boasts, coyly rear-ranging the folds of his white Scarlett O'Hara crinoline. "I like this dress; it frees me to wiggle. Twenty-four percent of all men show transvestism; it was in the *New York Times*. I took a shine to you. Did you hear my wife has terminal lupus?" His wife, greeting and seating guests, is an unassuming emaciated lady in gray ponytail and no makeup who looks better suited for organizing strawberry-picking outings with grandkids than parties for she-males. She's attended the fair for ten years. They have been married thirty-five.

He grew up in upper-class Georgia. After his confirmation, he woke up most nights with his mother's stockings on. He attended a military academy, got a Ph.D., worked for the U.N., and occasionally received packages of feminine clothes he didn't recall ordering and once found himself at a movie the-ater in a babushka. When he had a heart attack, a psychiatrist treated him for multiple personalities and urged him to "dress" consciously. His "madness" ended when he developed prostate cancer and was assigned hormones. "In our twenties, my wife and I were dogs in heat," he tells me happily. "In our thirties, the kids took up our time. In our forties, sex was great and, with menopause, we didn't have to worry. In the fifties and sixties, sex is companionship, being touched, and we give this to each other better as women. The estrogen neuters the penis so it hangs there dead."

The trophy for Miss Cinderella, "the most popular first-timer," goes to one of the Andrews Sisters, a colossal ruddy French maid in bobbysocks and red Oz pumps who fawns over the plaque he gets to hang in his garage. Miss Femininity is spindly and breakable, Miss Congeniality uncontrollably tear-ful. The winners give Oscar-style acceptance speeches thank-ing their loved ones, the organizers, and God, and recount tales of adversity, ugly male duckling to female swan morality tales. I watch the rigor of their suffering as they achingly move to the dais in their perilous heels and bandaged crotches, and

I know they don't value satisfied bodies but self-made ones. It's by strict method, attention, labor, and determination that men come to look like this. What they value is self-discipline and problem-solving, not tenderness. Femininity has become their philosopher's stone, the key to all the secrets people suspect are kept from them by invisible powers. They locate the American dream in every rhinestone they wear, every twist of their hips, every ghost of novel sensation.

At my table Melanie has been commiserating with a sportscaster in a mink about missing the Yankees game. "In the male world you always get access to sports," she complains. Her shaved chest pops out of her taffeta bodice as squeezed body fat; her wig is a petrified chignon; her smile, pasted on, gives her a prudish double chin. She has a ribbon on her Adam's apple, gloves, a gold-strap purse. She wants a TV, I want out, so we leave early. It's the last night, so we feel free to be graceless.

We find no sports bar on Commercial Street and Melanie acts obnoxiously, swinging her purse in one hand, her heels in the other à la *Dolce Vita,* emitting screechy, openmouthed, Brooklynese bimboisms ("Girlfriend, I swear!"). I decide to call it a night when she provocatively says, "I'm in a mood to do *anything.* Just name your desire." A cliché come-on. I say I want her to "undress" for me, which is against the FanFair rules. Her face drops. She stands up straighter. It's the final night, I explain; tomorrow she'll turn back into Mel. I want to witness this unveiling. Melanie is visibly disappointed, hurt that her disguise has "failed." I don't feel bad for her, because I don't think Melanie literally exists; I want to meet Mel because it's Mel I've talked to all along. I'd like to listen to Mel without enduring a voice that tries hard to sound insipid and a body language that crudely parodies my own. The show is over, I urge him again. Behind the smiling mask, his eyes look scared.

The voice gives in first. "Let's go to my room," someone I haven't heard before mutters. "I keep my promises." An hour later, a tall man comes out of Melanie's bathroom, blue-eyed, luscious-lipped, clear-skinned, muscled, and still moist, in crisp jeans and black T-shirt. He sits on the bed nervously and talks in a guttural professional voice about fatherhood: "I obsess on my existential issues, because of my daughters. But without my girls, I would be lost or back trying to have them. It's the cycle of the race. See, a female cross-dresser wants power; a male cross-dresser wants to be God, to appropriate the power of creation." I tell Mel he's just summarized all my views on cross-dressing. He asks me for my bra in exchange for his unveiling, as a souvenir. It's a useless old bra. I accept.

The next morning I feel relieved to return to a world where everyone is "genetic." Suddenly, even the excremental architecture of gas stations, chromium diners, and salt-eroded billboards looks reassuring. I stop at the first McDonald's and grin at some ordinary women in the parking lot chattering about relationships. Then I notice they're bony, lumpy, puffed-ankled, big-haired, and start to suspect they are men in drag. In the following weeks, these sightings increase. I recognize "CDs" everywhere—I sit by them in restaurants, pass them on the streets tottering shakily on stretched-out heels, glimpse their stony downturned faces under wigs in my neighborhood bar. Have my eyes been opened or distorted? I discover that my downstairs boutique sells fake breasts for $700 each, and the owner tells me he has a mailing list of half a million and FedExes to "the White House, the Supreme Court, the Pentagon." I find out I know artists who work part-time in salons like Alter Image "dressing" clients for $150 a session at lunch hour. The average customer, they tell me, is fifty-five, five feet eleven inches, 190 pounds, married. He arrives in a suit and asks to be made into a whore, prom date, stripper; the richest men want to be maids. Some clients also attend New York City's Finishing School for Boys Who Want to Be Girls, which offers classes for $375 or $2,500 and assigns homework such as "Creating Your Herstory." I'm leafing the week's *Newsweek* and stop at the picture of Erin Swenson, forty-nine-year-old divorced father of two, preacher, psychiatric chaplain, supervisor of seminarians at Emory University, Sunday school teacher, and marriage counselor, who has petitioned to retain the ordination she received as Eric; in a "historic vote," the Presbytery of Greater Atlanta upheld his ministry. Then I come upon a picture of myself in *Out* magazine, leaning against a tall cross-dresser in the crisp sunshine. The copy reads, "Giving realness to P-town's cross-dresser conference." Apparently the writers have outed me as a CD. It is *Out*'s only photo from the fair. I can't shake the premonition that I have entered the funhouse to stay.

New York:
Masters of Ceremony

"You'll find neither lock nor bolt to bound you, but loneli-
nesses will surround and hound you."

Goethe, Faust

*I left Provincetown with dozens of tapes and hundreds of pages
of notes, feeling overwhelmed. I didn't know then that I would
find no better way of conducting my investigation, because, with
people confessing away, I would be caught in the awe of their
catharsis and wouldn't know at what moment revelation would
come, so I would end up hearing many life stories and hugging
many strangers and would even grow used to the terror of sens-
ing myself at the edge of personal secrets no other had invaded
before. I decided to cast away all thoughts of sex in America
until I could devise a more efficient method of selecting my
material, and gave a poetry reading at St. Mark's Church. At
the typically dull reception that followed, I met a Columbia
undergraduate who knew my work and I mentioned my possible
new book and my surprise at meeting so many "normal" Americans at the cross-dressers' fair. Without missing a beat, she said
S/M was also full of normal and interesting folks and offered to
take me to her SoHo dominatrix the next day (she had an
appointment). I decided to let the answering machine pick up
her call and contact her after I had time to scout S/M clubs and*

see if my curiosity could be kindled. But she didn't only call, she came by my house, telling me to hurry up and get in her black BMW. So I met Psyche and her paying victims, and many others, and marveled at the sheer physical labor and intricacy of their lusts, all the while striving to quell my consciousness of being at the mercy of unconventional strangers. I became more adept at being both alert and meditative, at embracing the ambiguity and discomfort of my task, and even stopped knowing that I could be killed by any number of people whose extreme urges I'd blithely probed.

A Novice's Glossary

D/S (dominant/submissive) is the politically correct substitute for S/M (sadomasochist); top (sadist); bottom (masochist); vanilla (a nonsadomasochist); dom (dominatrix); slave (submissive who gives up all power in an S/M relationship on a twenty-four-hour-a-day basis); switch (enjoys both domination and submission roles); a scene (an individual session of any duration where the participants are in their S/M roles); the scene (the gamut of S/M activities and people referred to as a whole); B&D (bondage and discipline); edge play (dangerous B&D, such as electric cattle prods or asphyxia). Masochism, the tendency to derive pleasure from pain, traces its name to Leopold von Sacher-Masoch, a nineteenth-century Austro-Hungarian professor of history, whose writings on the subject are considered classic; he also composed the first published willing-slave contract signed by both S/M lovers. Sadism, the tendency to derive pleasure from inflicting pain, traces its name to the Marquis de Sade, who wrote famous classic works on the subject in eighteenth-century France.

n the heart of Manhattan's meatpacking district, where the wind off the Hudson blends with the stink of spilled cow's blood in sawdust, on a poorly paved and lit street with empty metal hooks hanging above it, one finds the unmarked entrance of a famed S/M club. When I first walk past the clothes-check clerk, following a quick pat-down and bag inspection, I come upon an extraordinary scene: a model-pretty dominatrix is slapping pounds of raw hamburger meat onto a pale, naked man, spraying him with ketchup, and grinding the meat into his own with her stiletto-heeled open-toed mules until he looks like a hideous traffic accident. The room smells of butchery. The dom, undeterred by the dead animal scent, finally stands up, her body squeezed into a sweaty hourglass by a rubber dress strapped open over her ass, and invites us to piss on him. A reedy man in a mask of mail, whose ankles are pierced so wide he could be hung from a meat hook by them, and whose muscular back bears twelve equidistant piercings tied together with leather string into a corset shape, obliges. Ice-T is singing "KKK Bitch."

A bystander tells me the "hamburger act" is inspired from Christian saints' massacres by hungry lions in the Colosseum; he points out another man who does "Spartacus on the cross." A St. Andrew's cross hangs in the corner next to a '77 Harley. "Spartacus," mustached and hairy-chested, looking like the Marlboro Man dressed in a leather penis cuff and eight rings around his testicles, is presently talking with a movie-stunts specialist about using explosives in his "scene." Hollywood seems grotesquely alive in this dank basement.

My new companion, watery-eyed and crisp, is a top-billed boxing referee, a Vietnam vet, and "the survivor of a beastly marriage." He tells me: "By treating humans like animals, I free the sexual animal in them. It's common sense. I knew I was S/M when I was four; I beat up kids because the sound my fists made on them turned me on." I tell him I don't quite understand the aesthetics of blood. "All beauty is made of blood," he preaches with a bare-toothed smile; "blood is life." He then breaks into a description of the traditional tortures for a suspected witch: flogging, scalding water, looking for the mark of Satan—the body part that had the kiss of Satan was supposed to be numb, so investigators put needles in the accused's body until they found a spot where pricking her didn't make her scream; if they didn't, they kept at it until she confessed; if they did, they hanged her. "I have a witch who won't confess," he proudly concludes, and leads me to a radiant queen-sized blonde in dog collar and waist cincher and needles through her nipples, lashed on a torture wheel. She hangs limply, breathing heavily. Convex ruby lines cross her belly, breasts, and thighs. "I'm a chubby chaser; I like my canvas big." He winks at me and generously offers me a go at her. I decline. "I took you for a top learning the ropes," he says, perplexed. "You aren't dressed for a slave. A switch?" Voyeur, I say, realizing the roles in this realm are painfully limited. Eager to initiate me into altitudes of pleasure, he showily pours watered alcohol on his quivering slave, announces, "I've come for you, my bride!" and sets her on fire. For a moment she is hidden by flailing tongues of blue flame. She screeches. The fire goes out fast and I smell burned hair. The stereo is playing Depeche Mode.

The torching draws a smatter of polite applause. My referee asks for a volunteer to put his penis in ice, then in a condom, and penetrate the witch. "In my first civilian job," he personably tells me, "I had an affair with my supervisor and beat her so bad she was hospitalized; I saw I had to learn how to inflict pain. In the S/M tribe our wisdom is handed down verbally from our elders. I took classes, apprenticed with a master. My motto is No Unintentional Pain. I owned a slave for nine years I practiced on. You'll need a master to study under; the guy you need to talk to is Roy; I'll give you his card."

Meanwhile, Spartacus's icy cock breaks into the "witch" in

a single, abrupt, dispirited surge. I watch her spasm. He smiles wickedly. "I'd come here to see what others were doing in the field and get inspired," the umpire prattles away in the manner of a busy conventioneer. "Now it's tame except on special party nights." Fridays are Slave Auction nights in the club; Sundays are N.Y. Jacks' jackoffs. On Shaved Pussy night, women who show a shaved pussy get in for free; on BBW Big Girl night, two-hundred-pound-and-up women get in for free; on Little Girl night, "schoolgirls" do the spanking. House rules forbid exchange of bodily fluids and alcohol consumption. This is sex as a spectator sport.

The place smells of urine, leather, mold, and dirt. Dozens of enormous men dressed as cops, soldiers, construction workers, or bikers posture about like show dogs. The mass of store-bought gear simulating machismo is sinisterly offputting; maleness is worn in effigy and fun, like a pawnshop war ribbon. It occurs to me that America's ethos of discipline and forbearance and bravado has come to this: the family man who nurses a lust for the whip, the businessman who yearns to be hung, the yuppie with a taste for piss. The Wild West mystique of the sudden quiet produced by a stranger's long-shaded entry into a bar of men anxious to do battle, measure their masculinities, and earn communal respect has been degraded to histrionic hyper-masculinity as a weekend stance. Primal tests (scarification, ingestion of bullets or piss) and codes of manhood, still extant in Appalachian burgs, urban ghettoes, and jails, are reduced here to brightly colored bandannas in back pockets that signal predilections. Right pocket indicates a submissive, left a dom-inant; blue worn on the left means cock-and-ball torturer; on the right, cock-and-ball torturee; red is for fister, yellow for pisser, green is for mercenary, brown for scat, gray for bondage, purple for piercing, white for novice, pink for tit-torture, black for pain, orange for anything goes. It's sex by code, with the geni-tals cuffed, chained, and subdued.

I estimate fifteen men to each woman, mostly stir-crazy

submissives on the prowl. Studies confirm what tonight's attendance shows: S/Ms are mostly men, and submissives outnumber dominants by ten to one. Women usually get introduced to S/M by male lovers, and find that the loss of control suits their socialization. Men discover S/M the same way they find bungee-jumping (originally an African initiation rite) or the men's liberation movement—in their quest to define masculinity in an egalitarian world. S/M provides a faux initiation ceremony: a public spanking or fistfuck under the guidance of an elder, followed by a hug or slap on the back, is a figurative affirmation of courage that shows the clan one is now a man. According to academic theorists, S/M is an "allegorical field" for normal transgression. According to the *Diagnostic and Statistical Manual for Psychiatric Disorders,* S/M is a mental disorder. According to the people who feel good when they hurt other people who feel good when they are hurt by other people, S/M is a seminal self-realization. "S/M makes me strong," Spartacus boasts to me in a telling string of clichés, "brave enough to withstand torture in patience. I'm a big boy; I got more balls than guys out there. We're all born into a world of suffering. We face death every day. No pain, no gain. You always hurt the one you love. What's life without pain?"

New York, with its choking accumulation of alert, discordant bodies crammed on a grimy isle, seems a natural greenhouse for compulsions that involve self-exposure and helplessness. The impersonal, forbidding city can induce in its denizens a sense of fatalism or worthlessness: there're always hundreds of people richer, prettier, more interesting than oneself, in plain view. The city also fosters exhibitionism: a fanatic commitment to survive and be noticed in the throng and appreciated.

The most mainstream New York City theme-park dungeon is The Vault. Admission is $40 for men, $50 for couples, $10 for women and TVs. The premises offer horse saddles, cattle-prods, suspension devices, a basement jail cell, and the requisite grunts, groans, sighs, sobs. Here the odor is of sweat and pine-cleaner. In the middle of the complex, idle guests— well-off tourists, men in suits, naked slaves, cross-dressers— sip sodas on couches or in empty cages, gaze at videos of tortures, and talk of Monday Night Football and fly rods. The bartenders are topless and unsmiling. A clutch of pudenda-flashing middle-management types compare canes, nodding gravely, as I stand at the bar, glass of orange juice in hand, watching an old master painstakingly immobilize a red-ball-gagged and earplugged slave with a spidery web of ropes; when he's done, he listlessly whips her thighs, causing her pelvis to rock against the ropes as if against a lover. But her pleasure doesn't seem to be the issue: her orgasm confirms the success of his domination, demonstrates his power and his technique, and proves that he is a master of the means of pro-duction of pleasure. In and of herself, without her pain, she doesn't exist.

A heavily eyelined mistress in a half-shaved Mohawk, leather hiphuggers, and a jacket with holes over her nipples checks me out with a "Don't fuck with me" air and barks, in an outer borough rasp, "You're looking at a lady, girl, lower your eyes." Do get off it, I reply. It works. "I get *paid* by these losers to beat them up," she confides, trading her bellicose tone for a sisterly one, still sounding like the young Jerry Lewis. "I rec-ommend it as the perfect relationship with a man. An hour or two and they're out of our life." To illustrate her point, she recruits a volunteer from the audience, ogles him disapprov-ingly, pinches his nipples to test his pain threshold, orders him to his knees, and applies a paddle. She soon sits on a chair and turns him into her footstool, hitting him indifferently, pausing to tighten the fastenings around his balls. A few onlookers jerk off in dim corners. He counts each blow with the yell, "Oh God, have mercy, Mistress!"

Men, some hooded, are strolling hungrily, mumbling indig-nities they want performed on them. Shawn, a commercial pilot in heels and apron, offers himself to me as a slave. "I'd love to lick your tiles clean," he baits me—a great come-on line for the nineties. "The ideal mistress is never pleased," he adds, standing at military attention, showing off his S/M scars. Shawn is proud to bear "marks from the battlefield of lust." "I've been beaten with a mace. One time a sloppy pro used a cat-o'-nine-tails of dog-collar chains that gave me scabs for months—earned me a reputation," he brags. He tells me what got him into S/M was the advent of AIDS.

AIDS is credited for the proliferation of paraphilias among America's middle class. Experts first sanctioned light S/M in the eighties as an alternative to risky sex because it does not require penetration or the exchange of fluids. In *The New Joy of Sex*, Dr. Alex Comfort lists "loving" S/M as a healthy variation; Dr. Ruth takes a benevolent view of spanking and bondage "as long as nobody gets hurt." Because most S/M deals with stereotypes in "scenes" less impulsive than the Sunday sex of an average couple, S/M has come to be seen as a harmless acting out of primitive psychic themes and a fantasy sport for aging baby boomers. This is the "demise of casual sex" predicted in the wake of the AIDS panic: safe-sex orgies in which genital contact is replaced by role-playing and where the byword is "consensual," positing volition as the crucial differentiating factor between getting clobbered and getting clobbered for pleasure.

Forced sex, such as bondage play, is Americans' top-reported fantasy in current research studies. The Kinsey Institute estimates that 50 percent of middle- and upper-middle-class Americans have tried bondage, 40 percent have experimented with S/M, and 5 to 10 percent engage in S/M for sexual pleasure regularly. These are more people than ever attended the Colosseum or Gilles de Rais's orgies. They are people raised on *The Little Mermaid* and happy-violent TV cartoons, who follow the directives of MTV and the fashion industry, buy Gucci stilettos and Versace bondage wear, read

Anne Rice or Linda Barlow, have seen *Silence of the Lambs, Tie Me Up, Roots,* and the publisher of *S/M News* on talk shows supplying his expert's opinion on mothers being spanked by their daughters' boyfriends; they may be patrician Junior League wives who host sex-toy demonstrations like the Tupperware ladies of old or teens who roam big-chain sex shops in malls, or romantic couples who weekend in bed-and-breakfasts that offer video cameras and fisting slings, or Wall Streeters who dine at La Nouvelle Justine, a New York City sports bar where the busboy-slave who cleans their table also licks their boots. In the nineties, torture has become a trendy back door to fevered consumerism.

"Outsiders are destroying S/M," Shawn complains bitterly, fiddling with his five-pound nipple clamp weights. "They just like to *look* liberated. They want costume drama. We lifestylers resent the New Age glitz and all the safe words and negotiations." "Safe words" refer to verbal codes devised to give a "bottom" control over the amount of pain endured. Whereas pleading for mercy is part of the act, a code word is an express request to stop. "Real S/M is a thrill, like having survived in battle," Shawn says, his face flushed with dismay. "If you want the truth, you got to meet this guy Roy I know."

Roy turns out to be a laid-back Maine native with thinning dirty-blond hair, sideburns, insecure blue eyes enlarged by spectacles, a Ph.D. in Colonial Lit., and aptitudes for making woodcuts of slave drawings, hunting with bow and arrow, collecting Puritan-era artifacts, and teaching "classic sadism." He's an S/M motivational speaker. He says things like, "My kit always contains five five-foot lengths, five ten-foot lengths, a twenty-footer, and two fifty-footers; I code my ropes by length, a trick of my dad's, who was in the Navy." Tops are the nuts-and-bolters of sex, the engineers. If we're all prisoners of sex (a misleading truism), they are prisoners of its hardware, at anachronistic odds with a world that values comfort over obedience, and nostalgic for a time when power was visible and social roles were assumed for life.

In a TriBeCa café, I ask Roy about the joys of topping. "I get a feeling of accomplishment," he says in a crinkly voice. "The rewards of a teacher. S/M is knowledge. I teach women their needs, the laws, rules, and rituals of their nature." I object that his S/M returns women to the position of property. "In the modern world, people are nonconsensually dominating and submitting all the time," he retorts, impressively self-aware; he's said all this before. "We're ruled by outside factors: clients, CEOs, suppliers. In sex I depend only on my tools I can test and retest. I'm in complete control to fail or succeed." This is not two people having sex, I say; this is intercourse as a contest in which only the man can lose, whose outcome depends solely on his competence. Roy upholds the tradition of an ironsmith who humiliates apprentices or a guild elder who stages gory tests of new members because he fears novelty. "This culture debases and emasculates *men*," Roy protests. "Look at the cover of *Newsweek:* it touts Viagra as the harbinger of the next sexual revolution." Like France's demoralized, impoverished nobles who developed Sadeian tastes, Roy uses his lovers as instruments to give him a semblance of the control the world doesn't offer most men anymore. I tell him replacing the phallus with ropes and tools seems to me an *admission* of fear and emasculation. His big face gets shiny. His eyes flash with distemper. "For an in-depth interview, you must let me tie you up," he says in a chilling, vitriolic tone. "We'll barter: your needs for mine." I try to talk him out of it, but my reasoning proves useless: I can find no common ground of reference. He implies I am a coward. With little respect for me left, he drops a note on the table with the phone numbers of his slaves and walks off.

Karen is a strikingly beautiful, studious nineteen-year-old Columbia sophomore who visits commercial dungeons, conscientiously saving her weekly allowance for the $200 half-hour fee. Short of masturbation, she's never had any other sex. "I'm a Christian," she explains righteously. "I won't submit to the whims of a Y chromosome with a tan." Her catalytic S/M inspiration was the *Village Voice;* she masturbated to the D/S personals until she gathered the courage to call advertised houses of domination, chose the most expensive as the safest, and made an appointment. She was sixteen. "I was lucky my age and gender got the attention of the headmistress. I was treated with kid gloves. I could go for free if I let a client play with me, but I'm very private and I'd never trust my body to an amateur." I wonder if this is the future of sex: an impersonal service only performed by certified specialists—a kind of massage. "I'm happy with my mistress. I'm untormented and free to concentrate on my work, and I'm sexually fulfilled."

She picks me up in a BMW, dressed in Jil Sander. On our way to meet her dom ("the best society dom in the U.S."), she quotes Irigaray and Kristeva and says that "at the end of *Gender Trouble,* Judith Butler explains that only violence can make the body 'real' anymore." Karen may be the feminist, and Christian, of the future. She says: "Being submissive puts chains on my body, but it releases my soul from bondage. I'm stronger than my vanilla sisters. S/M is a higher moral ground. My dom removes my imperfections. I am redeemed by every stroke of the lash. S/M is like having faith in God. All of my religious upbringing leads me to accept its truth."

At a Greenwich Village historical brick building we pass through a metal detector and face a short muscular woman in her fifties with pulled-back hair, a black fishtail dress, combat boots, and seamed stockings. She tells me to change her name to Psyche because "it's still illegal to treat a minor." Her firm no-nonsense approach reminds me of my school headmistress, a hirsute spinster with a weakness for the ruler and an ambition to teach calculus to third graders. Psyche strikes me as the self-conscious postmodern incarnation of that extinct disciplinarian.

"Psyche is all about love," Karen whispers circumspectly (I hope in euphemism); Psyche pops a Hershey's Kiss in Karen's mouth with a gesture of communion and sends her off. "S/M heals," Psyche lectures me, leading me deeper into shadowy corridors. "As I bring a whip down on flesh, I bring a soul to integration. I call it a faith experience. Patriarchal religions took our trust away from each other and placed it on God. With S/M, instead of putting your faith in God, you give it to another human."

Psyche's computerized client list has over three thousand names; 70 percent are lawyers ("Attorneys work with power and manipulation and don't know how to give it up without help"), followed by bankers and politicians. Ninety-nine percent are men, 95 percent married. Before they can be accepted, they are screened—police records, financial records, social security and credit checks—by Psyche's accounting wing. Most are treated by one of her "companions," who is selected from a scrapbook, along with a scene, during the $70 consultation session. Psyche mostly travels giving workshops, attending S/M balls and trade shows, and she's on worldwide outcall. Like a film director, Psyche's main job is to stage psychodramas and mind games. Her portfolio offers corporal punishments in Colonial jails, in an 1800s reformatory, on a plantation, on an English estate for offenses of manor or manner, in a medical exam room, in a Bible sect, at home by a stepmother; kidnappings and interrogations by Arab terrorists, mercenary soldiers, survivalists, skinheads, cannibals, the Inquisition, the KGB. Less imaginative clients keep diaries recording their common failings ("tardiness, clutter, being argumentative, forgetful, overspending, breaking valuables, bending a fender") and pay to be punished for them. Some clients have gone to her steadily for fifteen years.

"I will allow you a glimpse," she decides in her haughty, condescending monotone, leading me on through the gothic maze, "if you remain absolutely quiet and stern." She describes the client we're going to see: "Verbal humiliation and electrical genitorture interrogations. He likes to be a hero, but he can't go home to his wife with welts." She says he is a curator for one of the nation's greatest museums and has his own penthouse, Hamptons home, yacht. "Let's terrorize the establishment," she intones harshly, opening a side door.

The man is conventionally handsome. His nails are manicured, his hair tastefully highlighted. His lonely nudity stands out in the spartan, walnut-floored, mirrored room and discomforts me. "It bores me to humiliate him," Psyche says by way of introduction, with a derisive laugh her clients reportedly prize. "Pay me tribute, sissy-slime," she snaps, putting on leather gloves. He hands her three new C-notes, eyes down. In exchange, she throws him a needle-lined restraint jockstrap. "Put it on, leech, and await your examiner." "Mistress, may I speak?" he asks in a bland obsequious voice, dropping to his knees. I surmise he's accountably worried about my outside-world presence that Psyche has sprung on him as an impromptu humiliation. His clean-shaven cheek touches her boot. "You may not, shit!" she howls as we triumphantly stomp off.

Most submissive men are achievers who feel overburdened by social responsibilities (toward wives, children, employees, shareholders, patients) but are loath to delegate their power. They may spend $60,000 a year to find release from their tensions in torturing their manhood behind closed doors. Paying to be abused when and as they want to be, by visiting dungeons on their lunch hours or summoning doms to their offices to act out scripts they compose, they retain control. By allowing themselves to enter servitude, they defy societal expectations and feel a temporary liberation. When they don't even have to get an erection or to give a partner an orgasm, when they are dependent, trussed, and trapped, they feel happy; their pleasure is located in temporary self-erasure—in an enactment of death.

The best doms are female phallocrats who serve this masculine sexual economy as experts at caning, mummification, suffocation, "altered states," and, always, CPR; bondage alone is divided into "tie and tease," heavy leather, rubber, genital, Japanese rope, macramé square or slipped knot, Sweet Gwendoline, bondage sculpture, suspension, sensory deprivation, and so on. Middle-of-the-road doms, such as those in the *Domination Directory International*, are mostly ex-strippers or call girls with accumulated resentment toward men, who eventually turn to S/M because slaves like older women who represent mother figures, even obese, demonic-looking women before whom they can feel helpless. Doms don't have to smile, say yes, be touched or even looked at. Many adopt S/M in private and get a live-in slave, unable to deny themselves the comfort of a man who will scrub the toilet with a toothbrush and fix the sink and get hard doing it and still want to be called an insignificant worm. Unlike male tops, straight women get into "dom space" not because they're power-hungry but because they like it when men put them on a pedestal. Some even find their power oppressive or feel guilty. It's not easy to beat the hell out of an elderly man and have him call ten times afterward to thank them. But demand is growing: PONY (Prostitutes of New York) reports that intercourse, the most commonly requested service until 1980, has been replaced by S/M performed on the client as today's top preference. Smart hookers now gross $1,000 a week as doms.

Mistress Leah is such a converted professional. A "glam dom," vigorous and athletic, with impish eyes and the style of Louise Brooks, she works out of her home and pays taxes. An Orthodox Jew pays her to subject him to Nazi tortures; a banker pays her to piss on his wallet before which he kneels naked; a company boss pays her to be the company boss and punish him for embezzling. When I visit her, she's wrapping a dapper middle-aged corporate executive named Doug with Saran Wrap. It takes her over two hours and a dozen rolls to swathe him. "All my clients are grateful and respectful," she chats to me while her agile strong hands, gloved in latex, work without pause. "I'm not mass-marketed: I've no 900 line, no Web page, no video. I don't do phone sessions. A dom in the Upper West Side was found shot in her dungeon last month; I've never had a harasser." "I've got plenty of time today," Doug mumbles hastily, his diction feeble from constriction. "My wife is picking up the kids." Doug has been buried in wet concrete, glue, marsh, and bogs. He found constriction when he was given a body wrap at a mud spa to lose weight and got aroused. He now raises the ante each time.

"It's spiritual," he croaks as Leah wraps his toneless torso. "It helps me stay calm and overcome my need to move around. I learn acceptance. I will myself into another consciousness. In captivity, I go into a heightened state; I come out feeling like a butterfly." "Be quiet or I'll tear your tongue out," Leah admonishes, immobilizing his head in an inflatable hood with a breathing tube. He lies like a dozing, bandaged seal. She secures the wrap with electrical tape, hoists her mummified creation off the floor with winches and suspends him upside down. "I see myself as a sex educator," Leah says. "At the end of this, he'll run home and fuck his wife."

While Doug dangles overhead like a giant bat, she unlaces her boots and makes tea. I ask if domination reinforces the "woman as voracious virago" cliché. We sit on flogging stools and balance our teacups on a bondage table with hooks on the sides to fasten lacings and a lid that opens for sensory deprivation. Leah, sitting unflappably composed, tells me, "Domination is feminism. I was raised in a materialistic household. My mom had four husbands, all lawyers, very prissy and proper. I was a nice Jewish girl who knew nothing about sex. In college I worked as a model, a stripper, even a call girl, as my secret rebellion. I still had no personality, I was a walking coma attached to a TV. Then I took an S/M class at Eulenspiegel and it was like I saw the light. In my own life, S/M has brought me enlightenment and marital unity. If I wasn't a top, I'd turn back into a vegetable." Leah is married to a submissive travel agent. "We're into health, cooking, travel, exercise. Our S/M roles symbolize the union of opposites that is perfection." S/M devotees consistently bring up this creed: pain is good for the soul. And as people progress in S/M, their sex is less likely to end in orgasm and intercourse is reserved for procreation.

Because its erotic euphoria is tinged with religious zealotry, today's S/M fad reminds me of a spiritual movement that swept across Europe at another chiliastic age: the surge of penitential scourging in the fourteenth century. The outbreak of the plague in 1259 had inspired the first public flagellants. Soon, nobles and peasants led by bishops and monks whipped themselves in naked processions with scourges of knotted leather thongs; sins were confessed, follies renounced, people readied for a new spiritual life. From Italy the contagion spread to Germany, Hungary, Bavaria, France; in 1349 the brotherhood of flagellants was formed upon another outburst of the Black Death. Members vowed to obey a captain and scourged themselves twice a day for thirty-three days until their souls were free of stain. They marched through cities spreading the plague they were striving to exorcise.

The mass psychology that animated the flagellant hysteria resembles the current S/M notion of spiritual catharsis. The earlier, more marginalized and mostly gay S/M scene was hit first and hardest by the AIDS epidemic, so its nascent spirituality may be a direct reaction to the "scourge." S/M traces itself to religious (fetishistic) rituals of punishment and redemption, trial and reward. S/M is a symbolic exorcism of the reality of pain and mortality through a strict, sterile ritualistic reenactment. It's sex as atonement for sin. In that sense, S/M is sex mutated into Christian dogma, and its resurgence may stem from a similar impulse as the impulse refueling the revival of fundamentalism.

• • •

Ted and Stef are married lawyers who live in a luxurious, gated, New Jersey bedroom community. Their 6,500-sqare-foot house showcases prominent photos of their scrubbed blond children—ages four, six, and ten—silvered-copper furniture, murano glass doorknobs, and Hockneys on copper-leafed walls. Balinese music twangs through hidden speakers. "The kids are at Grandma's—normally we keep the den locked," Stef explains, offering me a tray of sushi. "We avoid the clubs because of our professional image, so this is the best we can do. We do hope you'll participate. S/M is a great icebreaker." The thirty or so members of Stef and Ted's social group are introduced to me, first names only. They arrive in sweats and carry their outfits in brown paper bags. After they change, we gather near a marble table bearing sake, wine, scotch, and dainty hors d'oeuvres. The doors are promptly locked.

Men smoke cigars and sip single-malt, women munch, and slaves fidget. Except for a sober-looking girl of twenty and a robust sixty-year-old professor who's been "in the scene forty years, since its inception," most guests are in their forties, dressed in costly vests, corsets, catsuits, and cumbersome heels that sink in the plush carpet. Some full-breasted women like Stef are naked from the waist up.

Male submissives gather about me like street urchins and ask: "You'll write about us?" A pushy collared slave named Max recites a life story everyone's heard before: "I was a sickly kid. I'd lie in bed and rub against the sheets to turn my pain to orgasm. I read of the Stations of the Cross and Jesus whipping the money changers and wanted to be a martyr; when the rest of the family was watching TV, I was in the bathroom whacking myself with a Ping-Pong paddle. This endurance made me less of a nerd. In college I went to S/M farms and built a dungeon, but it all felt fake until I met my wife. It was a relationship with a man she'd never dreamed of—a gender demolition. I'm her houseboy. She decides where I sleep, what I eat, where I eat, if

I eat, everything. We fuck with her on top in a strap-on; I like being penetrated more than she does. We've been monogamous sixteen years and have a contract like Sacher-Masoch's for life. She owns me, which is a tremendous responsibility for her." Is she the breadwinner? "She does my payroll, taxes, and trains rottweilers. I'm an eye surgeon. At work I'm a tyrant. It sounds like a split personality, but it's perfectly balanced." He is a fine-boned man with a neatly trimmed beard and unemotional, watchful, doctor's eyes. "Trust me, I've had decades of therapy on this."

At his leash's end, I overhear his wife say to other wives holding leashes: "I put him in collar and jockstrap and had him on all fours chase the ball, pick it up in his mouth, and put it at my feet. The kids were laughing. It's good discipline for them. Next time he misbehaves, I'll take him on a dog walk round the block." I stand aghast, absolutely speechless at the education of those children. "S/M couples don't divorce," she tells me in her Betty Boop voice, noticing my recoil. She sweeps her hand to include everyone present. "We have achieved the American dream. More wives would see their dreams come true if they understood that men want to be overpowered—for the guys, it's a vacation." I mention Dick Morris, Clinton's powerful political guru who fell from grace when his call girl mistress revealed that he liked crawling around naked in a dog collar and barking, "Woof-woof!"

"My wife and I like strangulation," Max gossips on. "She chokes me as she comes. It produces a bond you never get in any other relationship; a huge trust. It's the ultimate intimacy." Do they ever fuck without violence? "In Mommy role, she has me eat formula in bottles. She read up on baby-men and bought me adult diapers and big pacifiers. I just love to operate in diapers," he chuckles absurdly.

Louis, another leashed slave, in leather cape and shaved scrotum, interrupts Max: "S/M is about going through fire and coming out a man. Your mistress is your platoon leader, your

S/M buddies your comrades. It's community. Submission is a desire to be special, significant. History used to be intense. We had things to die for. Now we have S/M. S/M is an act of courage, and courage is a natural heroin shot." Louis is a millionaire race-car aficionado, and a Salomon Brothers trader.

I ask Stef how she got started in S/M. "Ted introduced me to it," she says with a blissful smile. "I met him at a conference; no man had captivated me like that. A month after our first date, I was wearing his diamond rings through my labia. Me! I was never so at peace. I swooned into his arms and stayed there." I ask Ted how *he* got into it. "Millions of years of social conditioning have made men the aggressors," he says quietly. "We're descended from men who raped. Consensual sex is new; it's not cool to say, but most women I know could use a heavy hand in bed." His mirthless laugh rings uneasily. "It's only role-playing," Stef enthuses with an enlightened tourist's smile. "I feel sexy all day if Ted grabs his belt and spanks me in the morning before he goes to court. S/M frees me from shame and from the anxiety of having to orgasm. I was socialized to please men; bondage makes my desire to please irrelevant." She overcomes her Calvinism by punishing herself for her pleasure; she finds peace by being whipped into senselessness. I'd say she buys into repression wholeheartedly if she needs to be "forced" into sex. "This theory of S/M being the product of repression is hogwash," Ted retorts. "We laugh at repression; S/M is primal instinct, pure and raw."

Ted invites us to his den, coyly announcing, "The house safe word is 'rape.' " The den walls are black aluminum and lit with forty or more flickering candles. My hosts give me a tour of their state-of-the-art playground: racks, manacles, swings, an iron cage, an immobilizing fisting sling, a coffin with a steel lid, a "Black Maiden" sarcophagus embedded with blades. I wonder what effect this Bluebeard's forbidden room has on their children's imaginations.

The guests chirpily help themselves to pegboards of tools

and couple in tableaux. Max's wife shackles him to Colonial stocks and applies a bull's pizzle to his shuddering back; he lets out low growls and streams of Thank you, Mistress's. Her beatings are methodical, devoid of anger or passion or lust. Soon she glistens with sweat. She lashes his back, stomach, nipples. His eyes are bloodshot. No one flinches. No one coughs. It's like being in a theater or a church. He is shrieking as she inserts a dildo in his anus and stuffs the pizzle into his mouth; he kisses it. Then she muzzles him, the pizzle protruding from the breathing hole obscenely.

"Watch her technique," Roger, the sixty-year-old chemistry professor, whispers in my ear; he's already hog-tied his twenty-year-old date in knots and sealed her inside the coffin. "As the endorphins build, the cone of positive pain widens and the top gets more range. Tools matter less than technique. S/M is body jazz: I know where I go, but I improvise, extemporize, my way. It's like any work of art." He leaves momentarily and returns with the empty cheeseboard. "This makes a sublime splat," he says pedantically. "So do spatulas, flyswatters, mixers, vice grips, shoe stretchers; an egg opener is a cock ring, a rubber glove a hood." His crafty gray eyes watch to see if his words turn me on. "I travel the eastern seaboard conducting private sessions with women who want to submit to me. I learn from every exchange. But I don't do volume. My interest is strictly in algolagnia—the pleasure of pain. May I give you an honorary demonstration? You *have* to try it to write about it. I've won over many vanillas. S/M is like lab work, conducting a chemical experiment; especially with a vanilla." S/Ms are convinced we would all love sex their way if we were not too inhibited to admit our deepest desires. There is a rising wing-beat in my chest: I'm getting claustrophobic.

"You don't want to be hopelessly mired in your genitalism," Roger lectures. The laboring couples before us duly direct their sexual energies away from their aroused or idle genitals, which they carry like extra props they can use to re-create

63

bodily carnage, or embellish it. S/M directs the erotic impulse away from genital copulation, inoculating the original object of desire.

A pewter Buddha is burning floral incense. Philip Glass is on the stereo. Louis is giving head to his wife's boot; as she shoves the heel down his throat, he emits a muffled moan, like he's just entered a woman. "You're a wuss," she says. Stef prances around with a saddle on her back, her mouth bridled. If she slows down, Ted's riding crop flicks her nipples, making her skip like a skittish thoroughbred. The sight of this friendly panting spouse performing like a prize horse in a contest ring disturbs me. Ted mounts her, whips her ass more soundly, rubs his chaps on her skin, digs his stirrups into her hips, yanks her hair, yahoos, and rides her, smiling contentedly.

"If I put myself in your mind," Roger whispers, his voice beginning to drip with contempt, "you're thinking Ted Bundy. So, I'll let you have *my* submission." He pulls down his pants and lies on a saddle, presenting me with a withered butt. "Take your discomfort out on me." For a second, there is pregnant silence; everyone is watching me. I do want to silence his garrulous patter, and I don't want to seem hopelessly mired. I want to remain outside the grip of his authority, but his believer's logic co-opts me. So I finally pick up a red suede flogger from a nearby steel carousel. "Don't say another word," I order him in the chilly timbre I've heard tops use, "one sound from you and I stop." I aim at fat and endeavor to produce a steady rhythm of chastening stings and matching puffs of his breath. My palms get clammy, my mouth dry. The swish on his frail skins frightens me. The margin of error seems enormous. I am using a stranger as I have only used an inanimate object before—a mattress, a dusty rug, a TV set that won't work. I have no motive for this act. I must force all empathy out of my mind. I have no prejudice against temporary sexual objectification, but the encounter is not at all sexual. I feel very distant from this prone body I'm being "intimate" with. I don't feel any raw, pure primal instinct surging in my body. In fact I feel mitigated, replaceable. My own flesh is inconsequential, replaced by an insensible tool of pain activated only by my will to play God.

Back at my hotel room, I find Daphne in an underdressed heap outside my door, patiently waiting to talk to me about her enslavement. She informs me her impromptu visit has been ordered by Roy, her master. I suspect it angered him that I never called any of his slaves. Daphne combines the caring frumpy air of a nun and the flaunted ardor of a precocious adolescent. She's in her forties, with a plump capable body and a guileless clement expression. She apologizes for "not changing into vanilla clothing": she "wasn't told to." Even as I find my key, she's extolling Master Roy: "He's a lifeguard: he inspects dungeons to make sure things are done right. He's very serious: he'll only flog in ten-hour sessions. I've had many owners. I've been bartered and sold. He's the meanest, the most detached and paranoid. He's my life source." She leans against the wall, her body contorted in the anguish of not knowing how to *be* around me. I ask why her erogenous zones require increasing physical and mental abuse. "Pain is an acquired taste, like sushi. I am a pain slut. I've ended up in the hospital, like in *9 1/2 Weeks.* My therapist put me on drugs to decrease my sex drive. But sex and S/M are different. S/M is freedom." Her only freedom I can perceive is freedom to give up her freedom. How can slavery, a vilified custom, be an attractive lifestyle to her? "It's a safety net," she says. "Everybody saves themselves as they can. Master Roy is good at protecting himself. S/M guards him from his rage; people who are fragile, like fine china, need to protect themselves and not waver unstably from lamb to beast. Since 1987 he hasn't been able to have sex," she adds, suddenly changing tune in an outburst of dispirited defiance. "He doesn't *know* how to orgasm and trust; he's killed his feminine part. He's denying the soul. He's dead inside. There's beauty in that because there's intensity."

She sits on my bed and cries for a while, fists clenched. She wanted to cut her wrists today in the shower, she says, but she had to call Roy for permission and he didn't give it. "He sent me to *you*. But if I can menstruate, why can't I cut my wrists?" she asks in a simple twist of logic. "Men live outside themselves and don't understand. We women have to do what we need to stay alive. I talk to God about that. I made the decision to live with God. And that, too, was a mistake. I re-create my abuse to get control of the original act that left me powerless. My parents beat me. It's a terrible fact." I find her hazy, possibly endorphin-overdosed. "I'm giving birth to myself right now and it's excruciating. The body is not enough. That's why I beat it. The body is the seat of trauma. My master saves me from myself." Intense pain may erase her memories or fears, but it doesn't kill them, I suggest; if it did, she'd quit S/M when she healed. "Maybe I haven't found the right master yet. Anytime, Madame, I may serve you, I will do whatever I can. No one will ever know what you do in this room, you can do with me anything you want. Feel free to make good use of me," she recites humbly and sincerely, unyieldingly helpless, and crawls under the bedcovers. The hotel blanket quivers with her sobs. She begs me to let her stay. It all feels like a test, the critical moment when I find out who I am.

I pity her and I fear her, as if her weakness were infectious. I have no doubt that she was ordered to spend the night. I'd like to kick her out and sabotage her master's will, but I won't use the undeserved power she's passed on to me. She's preempted my hurting her by welcoming it, and by making me responsible for her very being. My pillow is wet with her tears. I can't send her off. I turn off the light and spend the night in the armchair, tortured by an irrational premonition that if I doze off, I will wake up to find a bloody corpse in my bed. It's Master Roy's unarousing revenge.

Pensacola: War in Peace

"I don't trust anything that bleeds for a week and doesn't die."

From the film In the Company of Men

As soon as I was back, a close relative called to tell me that her husband had just been dismissed from the Air Force for insubordination to a female superior and had gone for a drive in such distress he ran into a tree and was now lying in a hospital, at age twenty-four, paralyzed for life. I flew to Florida.

In the military hospital, I felt as if I'd never left S/M. Men showed me their wounds with pride and meticulously described military life in the terms slaves had used to depict S/M. They reminded me of guys who wounded themselves sexually to feel physically complete or to "reclaim" their bodies or socialization rituals. In the street, the female denizens of the small military town eerily resembled the cross-dressers I had met. I wondered if my mind was projecting the covert sexual signs to which I had become privy onto an unsuspecting world, or if the real world was opening up to me in all its interconnected libidinal confusion.

As I stayed on, I began to fathom the immense bureaucracies of the military and the boredom it breeds. One of the tasks my relative had me perform was to talk her husband's boss into authorizing some insurance papers. I met a composed, forth-

right man, distraught by the chain of events that had left his young ex-sergeant paralyzed. We got to talking about the military sex scandals in the news, I mentioned my writing, and he subtly implied he would give me the needed paperwork if I helped publicize the peril facing the military. He was convinced the crackdown on sex would lead to war and said I owed it to my country to help debunk the crisis. I felt no one was interested in one more exposé on sex in the military and I was ill-equipped for the task, but I complied and, amid the tragic circumstances, resumed my snooping. I felt blasted into overheated psychic landscapes immeasurably far from myself. I had not had the time to determine the structure of my work, or define my audience. My subject matter sought me out and aroused more emotions in others than it did in me. Their convictions swept me into their lives so unequivocally I practically forgot myself. I had never imagined I could intimately know so many strangers so fast or contend with so many sexual crises.

A Novice's Glossary

AFB (Air Force base); SEAL (a member of the select corps of the Navy's superfighters trained to use guerrilla tactics and undertake covert assignments in inhospitable environments); hell tour (a transfer to a line of combat); BUD/S (Basic Underwater Demolition/SEAL training course).

The Eglin AFB in Fort Walton Beach, Florida, doesn't look like a hotbed of sexual activity. It's the largest Air Force base in the United States, but it looks more akin to a retirement community than a warriors' township, or an Officer and Gentleman compound. It's a one-story, geometrically laid-out suburb. The sky is flat, the land dull and cheap, the lawns neatly shaved, the houses, modest, ecru, gingerbread-framed simulations of trailer homes. Today, two out of three military men are married. The U.S. military is the largest day-care provider in the world. It runs schools, movie theaters, department stores, banks, gas stations. The Officers Club advertises Mongolian BBQ or French buffet nights; the Enlisted Club offers karaoke, oldies, blues, rock and top, Friday disco. Conspicuous posters announce bingo doubles, bowling, dart and horseshoe contests, casino trips, talent shows, doll-crafting and framing classes. Big American cars cruise idly and drivers wave gallantly. People move and talk at a snail's pace, don't loiter, and discuss food, movies, getting laid, washing the car. They're men of action trapped in a static warp, denied action, who seem to suffer their isolation and obsolescence as an interior putrefaction.

Master Sgt. Sam Lizt is a Logistics Support Squadron first sergeant, a "shirt." A six-foot, hard-muscled, heavy-boned woman with cropped dark hair, freckled skin, and thick manly eyebrows, she is humorless, practical, short-tempered. She struts and talks like the prototypical Rambo commando. Her fatigues, strained around her body bulk, make her look externally constricted and internally inflated.

"My job is to resolve personal problems for my people," she barks with the explosive authority of a cult leader. She doesn't strike me as a likely person to go to with an intimate problem. "I counsel on postmilitary options, clarify policies and rumors, act as a sounding board for families and airmen in trouble. I get middle-of-the-night distress calls from the emergency room or the security police. I do all I can to not have to take one of my people to court-martial. Now with the sex blowout, it's hard to take care of my problems; it has become one thankless job."

In July 1997, for example, the Air Force decided to court-martial 2nd Lt. William Kite, a supervisor of police for the 509th Bomber Wing in Whiteman, Missouri, for dating a female airman on base. The potential prison term was fourteen years. Kite, who was decorated in the Gulf War, fell in love with an airman not in his chain of command who subsequently left the Air Force so they could marry. The base chaplain saw her visit Kite in the hospital when she was enlisted and, in an eerie iteration of medieval prosecutions, called for an investigation. Kite denied having a relationship with his wife while she was in the service, but, when confronted with records documenting their phone calls, he confessed. He was charged with making false official statements. At that same time, the chief of military justice at Fairchild, Washington, was merely reassigned to another base when he married an enlisted airman on his base. Also at that time, sailors aboard the aircraft carrier *Nimitz* were disciplined, for holding hands, with the same severity as sailors who were found fornicating in the air-intake ducts of an F-4's engine. Because of these inconsistencies, in July 1997, Defense Secretary William Cohen created a task force to clarify and streamline military rules on consensual adultery and fraternization. In July 1998, the results are still pending.

"Now the rules are up to the whim of the officer in your chain of command," Sam confirms. "Before this shake-up, you had to be real stupid or evil and screw up repeatedly to get kicked out for sex. The rules banning sex in the ranks were always there, but if it was consensual, we turned a blind eye. Adultery that got detected was handled with dignity—counseling, a warning, threat of transfer, and finally transfer. At worst, there was a fine or a reprimand. Now it can lead to trial or discharge." The new military's muscular Christian ethos sees adultery as civic deceit, and reinforces a monastic remedy: if the flesh is weak, the answer is stiffer discipline. In this climate, people like Kite lose everything: their punishment is banishment—a secular damnation. For people who have been in the military since their teens, to be cast out for a sexual infraction means to live in perpetual moral shame.

Sam's job was to hear confession and give absolution. Until

recently, she could send the sinners away with wise words and the military's version of the Hail Mary. "I see people have affairs every day," she says. "Work is our social center, so sexual attraction is inevitable on base. It doesn't affect their performance. Their squadron mates don't know. They only tell me when they try to get out of it and can't, or realize they made a mistake. So to me the idea that Kelly Flinn's behavior was a threat to national security is preposterous. The president is an adulterer, and it didn't stop *him* from being reelected." Sam is referring to Lt. Kelly Flinn, the first female B-52 pilot, whose fall from grace in May 1997 astounded the nation. The Air Force forced Flinn to accept a discharge to avoid being court-martialed for adultery and lying to investigators. Flinn had an affair with Marc Zigo, a civilian married to an airman in Pinot, North Dakota; it all came out when she was a witness against a lieutenant charged with sexual assault. She claimed Zigo had told her he was separated. What the public saw as an everyday failing the Air Force saw as an officer using the power of her office to take advantage of an enlisted person (the wife); it reasoned that an officer who breaks a sex rule on ground may be tempted to disobey orders while aloft, which in Flinn's case meant while flying a B-52 capable of carrying a nuclear payload equal to all the bombs dropped by all sides in all modern wars.

Would Sam go out with a subordinate? I ask. "No. I'm thick-skinned, I think like a guy, but I'd lose respect, and I can't risk that. I'm not in this for the sex. I'm twenty-eight years old and have a hundred sixty-five people working for me. Only thirty-one are women. I need to be off-limits. So sex doesn't interest me." For Sam, gender equality has come at the cost of any sexual life. It's a familiar bargain: the new gender freedoms are bridling the sexual freedoms of military men and women alike, and eroding the boundaries between private and public life.

• • •

"You put young men and women together in tight quarters for long hours and nothing can bar them from having sex," asserts Chief Master Sgt. Terry Peters, a twenty-year Air Force veteran in charge of an Operations Support Squadron. We're sitting in his windowless office in a dusty corner of a hangar on Hulburt Field, a base formally off-limits to prying civilians like me. "Tightening the rules won't help. It wasn't discrimination that kept women out, it was respect. Amazons had no breasts, no husbands, no dads. If the public didn't want sex among soldiers, it should not have sent us women. When gals first enlisted, we went mad. There's nothing like not having to leave the barracks for sex. That was the military's sixties—the golden days before the feminization of our defenses." Was all that sex consensual? "I never heard that word before Witchhook. But nobody was crying rape. In my experience, the woman doesn't exist who doesn't want it." Were the women equally eager? "They weren't prissy about sex. It's the media that turned them into crybabies."

"Witchhook" refers to the 1991 Tailhook convention scandal, during which six drunk Navy aviators pushed female colleagues through a clothes-tearing flesh-grabbing gauntlet. In the tradition of sailors bingeing onshore, the annual Tailhook symposium was an occasion for junior officers and admirals to mingle and party. Most female aviators embraced the swaggering culture of men whose death-defying daily routine earned them such perks, and partook in "belly shot" and "leg shave" rituals, where alcohol was lapped up from their navels and their legs were given a high shave. But Lt. Paula Coughlin, a helicopter pilot, felt "practically gang-raped" by the gauntlet. When her official complaints were ignored, she went to the press. The exposure of its winking cavalier attitude toward its raunchy rites disgraced the Navy. The guilty men's superiors resigned. The suicide of Navy Chief Michael Boorda in 1996 was seen as a result of the Navy's hounding by Congress. What the military learned from that lingering infamy was to respond to sexual scandals with quick and thorough manhunts meant to show the public its unwavering commitment to civilian moral standards. In its eagerness to atone, it criminalized lust.

The modern military suffers from the "Vietnam syndrome": the fear of losing an ideological battle against civilians who affect its policy and budgets. This is why a culture that long prepared men for battle by unconscionable means now condemns any "toleration of Stone Age attitudes about warriors returning from sea," in the words of Navy Secretary J. D. Howard. Because the Tailhook scandal broke out right after Anita Hill's televised congressional testimony that had put sexual harassment on the map, it was seen as a chance to right Hill's wrong. Because of Tailhook, Congresswoman Pat Schroeder of the House Armed Services Committee pushed to repeal the law excluding women from combat, arguing that equality was the only way to ensure that military women received respect in a combat-oriented, male-dominated culture, and a provision repealing the gender combat ban was added to a military-budget authorization bill.

What Schroeder and Congress failed to recognize was that the main reason for the growing sexual turmoil in the military has been the very induction of women into the warriors' ranks. Typically, a society's ethics are chiefly devised to protect its women from the potentially violent, territorial instincts of its men. Or inversely, its ethics serve to prevent women from unleashing their potentially illimitable, insurgent sexuality, which is at radical odds with the social injunction to monogamy and child-rearing. In any case, the old rule of thumb that restless young men could play around so long as daughters of good families stayed unharmed cannot apply in a coed military. A new code of sexual honor had to be devised, so the sex embargo emerged as a blanket response to integration. Only sex between single consenting adults of the same rank is grudgingly permitted now.

Even this means that 8 percent of America's new coed force is at any one time pregnant, therefore nondeployable. In the Gulf War, 39 of the 400 women aboard the U.S.S. *Eisenhower* and 36 of 360 women on the U.S.S. *Arcadia* were evacuated for pregnancy. In Bosnia, in 1995–96, a woman was evacuated every three days for pregnancy; many reportedly conceived to avoid "hell tours." Women make up 14 percent of today's military, and 20 to 25 percent of new recruits. Since 1994, when basic training merged, eighty thousand jobs have opened to women in positions formerly off-limits, like flying combat planes, launching missiles, commanding troops, serving on combat ships. And because recruiters lower the official standards in order to fill their female quotas, lax evaluation leads to the very problems with sexual harassment the military wants to stop. Insecure or unstable recruits fail to fend off advances or know the difference between what is consensual and what is coerced in a world where superiors are trained to give personally invasive orders and subordinates to blindly obey them. In this vicious cycle, the battle of the sexes has become the military's most urgent and costly peacetime conflict.

"In training, your instructor is like God," Terry fires back, "it's like high school. The girls gossip about sex and get crushes on the teachers and compete over who will go out with whom. That's why we need strong-minded, street-tough women, if we must have women at all. Every harassment scandal is a recruitment flaw. Sergeant Simpson's accusers were wimpy naive little sluts."

Staff Sgt. Delmar Simpson, a twelve-year Army veteran and reported "stickler for the rules," was convicted in April 1997 for raping and sodomizing six female recruits under his command at Maryland's Aberdeen Proving Ground. He was sentenced to twenty-five years in jail. His deputy commander, Capt. Derrick Robertson, was charged with rape, forcible sodomy, and obstruction of justice. All in all, the so-called "Aberdeen rape ring" involved nineteen rape victims. The commander in charge of the six drill sergeants who were, along with Simpson, accused of sexual misconduct and awaiting trials was suspended for failing to ensure a sex-abuse-free climate; fifteen noncoms were suspended. Some trainees went AWOL to escape the sergeants, and one tried to commit suicide.

Yet the victims' courtroom testimonies were fraught with ambiguities: one said she had encouraged Simpson's attention; another said she found him attractive; a twenty-one-year-old, whom Simpson was convicted of raping five times, said he didn't force her to have sex—she thought it might lead to a promotion; a twenty-three-year-old whom he was convicted of raping eight times testified that he asked if he could touch her and she said "I guess." One private testified that, when Simpson shoved his hand in her sweatpants, she grabbed his hand and told him to stop it. "It wasn't sexual harassment," she said; she didn't report the incident and he never bothered her again. Another private told Simpson she wasn't interested because he was her drill sergeant; he left her alone. The court documents revealed a world of multiple partners, sexual score-cards, STDs, public sex in the game or TV room or on field maneuvers, and trainees seducing superiors to get respect. Offenders came from every rank. But 80 percent of the victims were white, and 80 percent of the accused black. Subliminally, America shuddered with an old pre–civil rights terror.

Then in June 1997, Sgt. Maj. Gene McKinney, the most senior of the Army's 410,000 enlisted men, was accused of sexual harassment. McKinney, a decorated Vietnam vet and African-American role model in the Pentagon, was appointed to a commission reviewing the Army's sexual harassment policies; this outraged his former public-affairs secretary, Sgt. Maj. Brenda Hoster, who charged him in the media of sexual harassment. He was asked to retire. When five more women brought up similar charges, the Army held court-martial hearings. Hoster testified that McKinney made a fumbling pass at her in an Oahu hotel, telling her she aroused him. A Navy chief petty officer testified he offered to show her "passion like she'd never known." An Army recruiter said he asked if she wanted to kiss him ("Hell, no, that's the last thing I want," she'd replied). A sergeant recalled him saying, "Men, women, we have needs." For these laughable comments, which in the right romantic circumstances might even be charming, McKinney faced fifty-six years in prison. Even after a military jury cleared McKinney of all sex-related charges in April 1998 (except for a count of suborning perjury for telephoning a witness), his career ended, his pension was withheld, and the point was made that standard tacky flirting with uninterested women was a military crime.

McKinney's lawyer had threatened that, if convicted, his client would expose "the Army's dirty laundry" by showing that white officers who faced similar charges had not been prosecuted. McKinney, the first black to serve as sergeant major, called the allegations racially motivated and filed a motion claiming discriminatory prosecution. This clash between two long-excluded groups—blacks and women—anxious to protect their equal rights within the military has created an unexpected political ticking bomb. Cmdr. Robert Davis—who was accused of making sexually suggestive comments at a dance, was put in a psychiatric ward, was eventually cleared of all charges by a court-martial, and forced to retire—sued the Navy for discrimination, blaming his white commanding officer, Katharine Laughton, of racism. Capt. Everett Greene, slated to be the first black head of the SEALs, was also accused of making improper overtures to two white female subordinates while he was in charge of the Navy's office on sexual harassment, was also acquitted by court-martial, and lost his career. These racial tensions have further convoluted the issues of sexual harassment.

Yet the fact remains that thousands of military women are sexually assaulted every year—ten times more often than women outside the ranks. Confidential Army case files revealed that women soldiers had been raped in their rooms, during showers, on field maneuvers, often at gunpoint, and Pentagon surveys showed that three-quarters of the women polled reported some sexual harassment. In September 1997, the Army released its largest study of sexual harassment; the ten-month review concluded that "sexual harassment is commonplace. . . . Soldiers seem to accept such behaviors as a normal part of Army life." The survey revealed that 78 percent of women and 76 percent of men reviewed had experienced "crude or offensive behavior" in 1997, the year of the military's crackdown on sexual misbehavior; 72 percent of women and 63 percent of men had known "sexist" behavior; 47 percent of women and 30 percent of men had received "unwanted sexual attention"; 15 percent of women and 8 percent of men had experienced "sexual coercion," and 7 percent of women and 6 percent of men "sexual assault." The two-volume study noted that the Army's attempts to educate its ranks are a failure; the ranks still have little understanding of sexual harassment and how to combat it, and as a result they "uniformly do not have trust and confidence in their leaders." To alleviate the "breakdowns in human relationships," the Army pledged to add more chaplains and a hundred new lieutenants to training units to give company commanders time to deal with ethical issues, and to put a three-star general in charge of overseeing moral training—to intensify all the usual cures that haven't worked up to now.

In November 1996, the Army set up a sexual harassment hot line in the wake of Aberdeen; it received 3,930 calls in the first week, for grievances dating back to World War II; 506 of the accused were turned to the Army Criminal Investigation Command, including 10 chaplains, 13 drill sergeants at Fort Leonard Wood, and 5 sergeants at Fort Sam Houston medic school. A concurrent Veterans Administration study found that 1 in 4 female veterans had been raped or sexually assaulted on duty. The VA opened sixty-nine centers to treat these victims—some five thousand women—for post-traumatic stress syndrome (psychologists liken sexual abuse symptoms to battle trauma). And during the Gulf War, sexual assaults ranged from an overnight guard who awakened to find her mate fondling her to a twenty-one-year-old private being raped at knifepoint by a sergeant. No doubt, wartime rape is a grave matter. These violations of fellow soldiers in ways reserved for the enemy could ostensibly qualify as treason.

This is why an institution dedicated to physical fitness and aggressive readiness, which uses humanity's animal elements as its raw material, has come to suppress its members' sex instincts as doggedly as religion once did. "We relaxed the rules too much," announced Gen. Dennis Reimer, the Army chief of staff, post-Aberdeen. "The goal is to desexualize the environment as much as we can." But can the Pentagon suppress the instinct for rough sex without suppressing the instinct to kill?

In June 1995, two SEAL buddies, Billy Joe Brown and Dusty Turner, were sentenced to life in prison for kidnapping, molesting, and killing eighteen-year-old Jennifer Evans in Virginia Beach near the Little Creek Amphibious Naval Base. They'd rendered Evans unconscious in thirty seconds with a SEAL maneuver. Before Evans, with whom they'd wanted a three-way, they had shared various women whom they brought to the barracks and gang-banged in front of their teammates. "It's a camaraderie thing," Turner told *Details* magazine. "You do everything else together. You sleep, eat, shit, together." "You've so much frustration, you need to release it," Brown added. "Half the guys are into group sex," a teammate continued. "If they decided to relieve of duty all SEALs who lived as Billy and Dusty, there would be no SEAL teams. SEALs are people who must do extraordinary things, and unfortunately that means knocking a few bolts loose." Brown's BUD/S class had chanted rhymes about sliding curling irons into vaginas.

Young men assiduously trained to be killers cannot be lambs. Soon after, in September 1995, three American sailors again revealed to their nation the limitations of enforcing political correctness on its fighters when they raped a twelve-year-old Japanese girl on Okinawa. Richard Macke, the chief naval officer, joked that they should have hired a prostitute. By the end of the day, the comment had cost him his job. "We bring young men and women into the armed forces to be warriors, in a warrior culture," Gen. Colin Powell later told the *New Yorker*, trying to explain the schism between pressure groups in modern politics and old military habits, "not social workers."

"Whoever heard of an army afraid of sex?" Terry Peters asks me. "Being a member of the military is losing its meaning, its valor. The ideal of manhood is shot. The best guys are leaving because our Defense Department is run by civilians in the Armed Forces Committee sitting in a boardroom worrying over hanky-panky. The sex crackdown is self-defeat—self-assault, not sexual assault. We've become a guilty, condemned, defeated army." The graffiti in the dingy bathroom behind Terry's sunless office reads, "Die or Kill." Men aching for battle may unreasonably see rape as a kind of practice. And military rape has been around so long it is a deeply entrenched cliché: worldwide, soft-core pornography regularly disseminates images of "forced" sex and weaponry—such as naked women giving fellatio while lying on tanks or at gunpoint or straddling guns, popular images that are as old as the French Revolution. It's no wonder that, in times of peace, men treat rape as a substitute for war.

Arlene and I are huddled over a shiny tin table in the large protected space of the faux-ornate Enlisted Club, within the larger confinement of the Eglin base. Two miniature Filipino wives giggle with an officer at the next table, carpeted yards away. No one talks much. Most patrons watch the surround-sound TV, deeply and mindlessly involved in the illusion of drama and fast pace. They are peacetime military people: indifferent to autonomy, happy to have all necessities taken care of, used to ACs, microwaves, packaged foods, sweats, waiting lists, signing up and getting authorized for the simplest tasks. The military shelters them from the dark, flawed world out there, much like the Church protects its priests. Their lives, like their homes and uniforms, are prefabricated, automatonic; their shared aesthetic is camouflage: hiding everything individual, in the name of national security.

Arlene is a senior airman who joined with the dream of being a Kelly Flinn, but failed the flying tests. She is consoled by her new Purple Heart, which she got for laceration wounds suffered during a terrorist bombing in Dhahran, Saudi Arabia, in June 1996. She lives in the dorm, eats junk food, sleeps twelve hours a day, makes $20,000 a year, and manages to save money. She doesn't have a "serious" boyfriend, because the parameters for a romantic relationship on base are too nebulous, and everyone she's ever met in town is associated with the military. She is twenty-two, blond, ponytailed, still prone to teenisms, bubbly, and good-natured. Her tall angular body gives off a stout sexual odor.

"We've become segregated," she eagerly complains in a girlish voice. "This harassment thing pits us against the guys. The guys think the scandals are our fault and look down on us. They blame us, even though we suffer from it the same. When I was first stationed in England and Germany, it was *Animal House*." Arlene is an Army brat. "There were no virgins over the age of twelve in any base we lived on," she explains. "We had nothing else to amuse ourselves with. We slept with the kids we baby-sat. At twelve I slept with a boy from school at lunch break all year. Half of us kids enlisted. None of us would stay in the force if we had to give up all sex. Sex isn't about taking orders." But the new tough moral regulations are meant to protect women like her, I say. "My mother had me when she was fourteen," Arlene says. "I have four dads. The military gave me purpose and independence. Now sexual harassment is ruining it for me. I think sex harassment is too general. It includes looks, gestures, letters, calls, teasing, whistling. Words aren't rape. I've never seen anyone lay his hands on a girl on the job. At the club I've had gropes and derogatory words. I get them from construction guys on the street, too. Men get their equal share of come-ons from us. I've told a guy I wanted to goose him, point-blank. I grab guys' balls. And we always talk about sex at work to pass the time, especially girls do, because men are scared now. But if someone bothers me, I tell him off. I don't need help."

Our murky legal doctrine of sexual harassment came into being in 1964 in a last-minute amendment to the Civil Rights Act filed by conservative southern congressmen trying to kill, and mock, that bill. It was not debated or enforced until 1977, when Catherine McKinnon convinced a Washington district court to award damages to a woman whose employer retaliated for her refusal to sleep with him. Until then, courts had ruled that sexual overtures in the workplace were "personal" and didn't constitute sex discrimination. McKinnon read the amendment as referring to quid pro quo "put out or get out" cases that created a hostile work environment, and even argued that, in patriarchy, any woman's consent to sex is inherently coerced (implying that there is no sex free of harassment). The general public was introduced to it in 1991 during the Clarence Thomas congressional hearings. Thomas's alleged requests for dates and distasteful office banter came to redefine *sexual* harassment; more emphasis was placed on the grossness of his conduct than on its impact on Hill's ability to work, because the Republicans who sponsored his nomination to the Supreme Court found it more expedient not to quibble on the definition of sexual harassment, but to exonerate Thomas from a personal stain by attacking Hill's version of the facts. Since then, the courts have broadened the definitions of a hostile work environment; in 1998, the Supreme Court awarded damages to Kimberly Ellerth, who filed for harassment after quitting her job when a vice president made sexual advances at her, although she didn't submit to them, didn't complain at the time, and didn't suffer any untoward consequences for refusing them. This puritanical interpretation has spawned a punitive climate where companies, agencies, colleges, and busybodies police consensual sex as the Church once had.

"Forty thousand women served in the Gulf," Arlene goes on. "People had sex in tents, latrines, Humvees, everywhere we could; but we were a team first, and we just had sex when we had nothing else to do. We were not that watched then." I ask if there was any S/M, golden showers, or other kink. "No. I saw a lesbian fling and maybe there was anal sex. But we had danger outside. Sex was the safe part. I don't think there's any kink in the military. We're real straight and disciplined."

During sex, Arlene often visualizes herself flying a B-52 across enemy fire. She thinks war is an aphrodisiac. "Falling bombs are kind of orgasmic," she describes. She arches her back and stretches her legs in what look to me like reflexive mating signals. "Once you hear an explosion and feel the ground shake and watch the blast, you never forget it. I've had sex during bombings and it's the best." I say it strikes me as perverse that the ethics of bombing children are discussed less in our society than the ethics of making out in an underground shelter while bombs fall all around. I think sex in the circumstances Arlene describes is a resistance to destruction, an act of life amid slaughter—the opposite instinct to the one spurring warriors to disseminate missiles.

"I think this crackdown isn't really about sex," Arlene argues. "We're nonessential because of budget cuts, we're overstuffed, and sex is the excuse. If they can't get you on anything else, they know they can get you on sex because everyone has sex in the military. They want us out. They let us off with voluntary separation incentive pay; and they keep recruiting. My job starts six hours after I get in, and even then the computer does most of it. We're like temps in a corporation. The Army has no honor anymore; it's false advertising." Realistically, the military requires a slave class for its continued existence; but American optimism denies the existence of such a class, so the military courts disaster if its slogans concerning the dignity of man wear thin. This is the impasse the modern military is groping uneasily to escape with remedies such as gender integration and forced chastity.

Chief Master Sgt. Terry Peters has thinning gray hair, a sharp nose, choleric eyes, a sloppy uniform—his jacket is too tight, his trousers not long enough. He's given himself a coffee break and is sipping his beer at the Aero Club in a methodical rationing way, making it last. "Sex is the concession the brass is making to politicians who control our purse strings," he grumbles, fiddling anxiously with the controls of his tiny portable TV. "They're bartering our sexualities for weapons. Their scheme backfired, but they can't stop without losing face, so they up the pressure and hope it will die out. Sex won't die out. The Army will. We'll end up with pussywhipped soldiers, only because what makes sense in the field doesn't fly in D.C. The virus has spread up to the top generals."

After the gender wall came down, military men, accustomed to relieving stress by flirting with women who are fetishistically drawn to men in dress uniforms, found the women were now in uniform, too. This changed the power dynamics of casual machismo: sex threatened to unsettle the sacred order of power in the military. As the outsiders became insiders, the culture toughened its mores to protect its old structures. And men ironically began to be rewarded for their level of emasculation. In the formidable bureaucracy of the permanent peacetime military, a charge of sexual impropriety became an effective weapon to kill off a rival. The new prohibitions have fostered fear, gossip, and petty machinations, now that anyone can call an 800 number and ruin a venerated career. All this is transforming the proud warrior culture into a "he said, he tried, he gestured" public sideshow. Promising officers with sexually colorful histories leave the military to avoid risking defacement; those who stay, out of loyalty or need, must worry over who in their past may retroactively do them in, and forfeit their legal right to privacy.

In June 1997, Air Force general. Joseph Ralston was disqualified from candidacy for chairman of the Joint Chiefs of Staff when it was revealed that he had had an adulterous affair thirteen years earlier, when he was separated from his wife, with a woman who was not in the military. The offense seemed so harmless that Defense Secretary William Cohen tried to "draw a line" against "the frenzy of sexual allegations"; he was accused of double standards in view of Flinn's case. Ralston's career effectively ended. Ironically, in 1995, Ralston had signed an order to strip Lt. Gen. Thomas Griffith of his command of the 12th Air Force because of an adulterous affair Griffith had had with a civilian at a conference. These persecutions are no longer unusual, nor are they mere media blips; they are individual tragedies that also implicitly serve a greater social purpose: they warn the public away from an unruly thirst for sexual satisfaction and initiative. They are moral lessons meant to evoke pity and fear in the populace and to place its sturdiest and most precarious impulses under submission. A traditionally female disorder, hysteria, which consumed the Puritans in 1692, is sweeping across the "feminized" military, and, through the media, it is contaminating the nation.

"It's just a trade-off," Terry gripes. "The brass gives in on sex to get more money. But we spend the money to automate and make it easy for women, and cling to enormous weapons made for a war that never came, and don't train our forces for small wars. Gender-merging has our priorities screwed up. If we're called to fight, we'll be the laughingstock of the planet.

As it is, we'll need our nuclear force to avoid defeat. We're flirting with a nuclear apocalypse just to keep our soldiers from fucking hard." Terry is saying this: if the military is weakened, it may have to resort to nuclear power to win a conflict. The military refuses to let go of the warheads it maintains on hair-trigger or of its right to respond to a nonnuclear attack with nuclear power, despite the recommendations of the National Academy of Sciences and the secretary of defense; instead, the leadership accommodates other civilian demands, such as that for sexual equality, in order to appease its critics and protect its turf from the defects of democracy.

But in the unremittingly physical world of the military, sex differences are undeniable. The average woman has less height, upper-body strength, muscle mass, skeleton weight, aerobic capacity, and endurance stamina than the average man. Women don't meet the standards for 70 percent of the Army specialties. Female recruits are injured at twice the rate of male grunts. Drill sergeants find it hard to humiliate women—in a rite meant to break down the sanctity of one's person, eliminate the fear of shedding one's blood, and instill the sense that a soldier is the chattel of those he or she serves. In today's Navy, the women's obstacle courses take place indoors and runs and push-ups are not obligatory, whereas "integrity development seminars" are. In the Marines, fitness for women is tested by a flexed-arm hang instead of pull-ups, and half the number of sit-ups. And the Army has devised a costly Freshette Complete System, a portable contraption that enables women to pee standing up in the field.

These adjustments strike the men as unfair and contribute to the current decline in enlisting men, who, in addition, fear purges like Tailhook's where every aviator in the convention had to pass a "clearance scrub." These changes *incite* the sexual revenge of territorial male warriors, which inevitably leads the women to seek refuge from sex in the law, which further alienates women from the close-knit corps and makes them feel either guilty or like outcasts. Clearly, in the inarticulate military culture, the new sexual McCarthyism only compounds men's difficulties of understanding female sexuality. Besides, the laws that protect women from predatory men help perpetuate women's traditional positions as sexual casualties. Sexual harassment, designed to prevent gender discrimination in the workplace, preserves both the sexual objectification and the desexualization of women: it objectifies them by emphasizing the sexual aspect of their presence in an integrated environment, and desexualizes them by forcing them to be either frigid or victimized. In effect, it is an antisex law.

Since the disorder in the military is a result of gender integration, the bigger question remains why women are essential to the nation's defense. America does not need women's physical powers or numbers to maintain its stability. And integration can gravely affect wartime policy, so long as America is unprepared for the actuality of sending women to the front where they are vulnerable to rape and assault by the enemy. Wars can unreasonably escalate over lesser traumas than the mass molestation of female POWs. Despite these drawbacks, the military aggressively recruits women for ideological (what Terry dismissively calls feminist) reasons: to bolster its public image of gender blindness and moral authority.

The military may advertise itself as a provider of opportunity and experience, but that polish disguises a harsh reality of absolute obedience, a Faustian pact that requires the sacrifice of life and freedom. Women don't need to pee standing up or rape or bomb to be equal. And the military only moves them from the familial system of control to a new function of submission. Its flag-waving ideology neuters and "masculinizes" women, so that they may one day die for its preservation.

It is a familiar pattern. Women's economic and political freedoms have come with subtler, more cynical sexual controls: via politics, media, advertising, entertainment, and law the prevalent ideology coerces women into physical and carnal purity, conformity, uniformity. Female sexuality is still perceived as a preeminent threat to the social stability that America needs to defend itself against—even at the cost of sending women to do battle. This whole enterprise, from scandalmongering to scapegoating, strikes me as sexism in camouflage.

"Sex is about conquest," argues Terry Peters. He is playing Nintendo on his mini TV. At the last second he misses the takeoff ledge and "dies." He doesn't react. He just starts over. "I *like* air warfare," he says to the screen. "It's why I joined." The game is Space Griffin. His character is "Killer." "Sex is not just diversion," he adds. "Sex is a locking of horns, a test of will. Like war."

Throughout history, soldiering has been an expression of the young masculine task of confronting fear and expending wayward testosterone. The link between militarism and masculinism is pancultural. When a nation asks its men to dehumanize fellow humans into enemies, it implicitly permits their incivility to be extended to the savagery of rape, so long as its own women remain out of reach. Until the seventies, U.S. troops marched to the chant, "Two, four, six, eight, / Rape, kill, mutilate." The earliest hymn of the Bible, Deborah's song, is a war song, followed by the savage tale of how Benjamin's tribe got wives via rape (Judges 5–21). Deuteronomy gives more direct advice on the subject: "When the Lord [gives you a city]. . . you shall put all its males to the sword, but the women and the little ones . . . you shall take as booty for yourselves; and you shall enjoy the spoil of your enemies, which the Lord your God has given you" (20:12–15). The Roman Empire was founded on the mass rape of the Sabines. To this day, rape is a common war tactic, used—most recently in the civil wars in Africa and Bosnia—to psychologically defeat and agitate the enemy. And, when action is limited to mock-battle exercises, brutal sexual rites keep the barbaric instincts alive, and enhance the unity and collective ideology of a corps, typically to the denigration of women.

"We *need* to be brutes," Terry harangues, his feet on the metal table. "We didn't join a convent. The military is bodily work. Remove sex from it and you end up with eunuchs as your army. We *need* sex to stay fierce. Those who can't take the sex should get out; they're not made to be in an army. But if you say this stuff out loud, you're terminated with a black record. It's a left-wing conspiracy!" The desexualization of America's forces in the nineties has fostered anger, disappointment, and despair among the enlisted who see their repression as enfeebling the nation's defense and mocking its warriors. Men accumulate a mounting resentment for the women. As every barracks becomes an ideological battlement and every peer a potential sex-snitch, many find it hard to resist the sexist undertow. And bunker mentality spawns lynch mobs and coups.

Clearly, sexual coercion is repulsive. But the assumption that every woman is in a position of sexual weakness and needs to be protected discredits equality. And the loss of intimacy in the workplace, where we best know each other, dangerously limits the pool of available mates in our workaholic society. We don't want to live in a desensitized world where life at school, on the job, in the neighborhood, in the cafeteria, on base, on a daily basis, is robbed of spontaneous sensuality, where the human body is an apathetic, feared boundary. We now risk losing a vast dimension of existence: the body language through which women and men suggest and manifest wonder, tenderness, defiance, arousal, delight. Lust is not only a physical but a discursive urge, a wordless eloquence. Sex is about odds-making; ambiguity, as well as loss and hurt, are inherent in human relationships. The way we learn about, and improve on, our sexual relations is by trial and error.

"This inquisition will end when we have a war," Terry is saying, blunt as a stone, nuzzling his empty cup, keen to have the last word. "So we will. That's what we're paid for." We all know Helen of Troy's infidelity was just a ruse for Greek men bent on war. Wars and whores, as Aldous Huxley put it, battles and brothels, break all the rules. War is how rigid cultures regenerate. Periods like this one, when our myths of self-sufficiency, goodness, and safety are shattered end in unscripted ways. It is a disheartening state of affairs that, in our evolved age, war is seen by our warriors as the only way out of sexual repression. It should be alarming because, as Plato said, "only the dead have seen the end of war."

San Francisco:
Blood Simple Babes

"Some say thronging cavalry, some say foot soldiers, others say a fleet is the most beautiful of sights the dark earth offers, but I say it's whatever you love best."

Sappho, c. 600 B.C.

These days we tend to assume that the exposed life is equivalent to the examined or well-lived one. In our new ethic of media-ted self-revelation and easily wounded feelings, we use Holocaust-like terms such as victims *and* survivors *to describe people who have been lied to by lovers or groped by distant relatives. In the meantime, the rants of rancorous talk-radio hosts and talk-show guests, the numerous trivial tell-all memoirs and the egregious exhibitionism of Madonna's S/M, Rodman's cross-dressing, Anne Rice's vampirism, Ellen's sitcom lesbianism have unburdened consensual depravity of stigma, but also of meaningful individual resonance. Words and signs are displacing our genitals. Emancipation has brought us no peace.*

And because we are confronted by too many hyped sexual options and potential public accusations, risk-assessment now dictates our sex lives. What used to be the prison of modesty has become the brig of accountability. We live in fear, not of God, but of ourselves. This makes us prone to passivity, or to sloganeering. Eager to find some stability and coherence, we increasingly define ourselves by our sexual orientation. We code it in our clothes, our speech, our posture; it confers our community and our status. But by proclaiming ourselves a "lipstick bottom" or "leather top," we restrict our experience to the roles we invest our identities in. A bald butch dyke is as much a cliché today as a housewife. Even people who fetishize amputees or nail their own penises on planks have ready theories for their proclivities that sound eerily theological and unsexy. Support groups reinforce this sexual isolation, as do the doctors who medically alter the body to match our mental concept of our sex, and sexperts who suggest that sex can be treated and solved. The end result is that we still don't depend on our distinct psyches to define our sex lives, but on the ideology of a society that divides human sexuality into rigid categories in order to control it, and dresses it up as a cornucopia. In all these ways, sex is getting deeroticized.

I had gone to San Francisco to visit an old friend, a lesbian poet with the quick-moving, peremptory personality of a bull-fighter. When I told her I had been investigating S/M, she argued I did my gender an injustice if I ignored the "strong" women in S/M. She was firm and impassioned, urged me to change my ticket, and called up her S/M friends. Most were unwilling to talk to outsiders. She explained to them that I was not "media" and to me that she was taking a great risk on my behalf, since her friends would hold her responsible if I betrayed them. I couldn't see how liberated women could still live "closeted" under the fear of detection and rejection. In an effort to convince me, my friend effusively divulged the most secret details of her sex life. She had cut herself out of frustration and then rebellion as a teen, and later incorporated it into sex. I remember saying, "I know what you mean"; I could imagine a kind of ultimate erotic abandon that would climax in blood. But I didn't know what she meant until I saw the unmediated reality—what St. Thomas Aquinas calls "the authority of the senses."

Her friends were driven, well-spoken, well-read, familiar. Like most S/M fans, they craved both civilized discipline and maenadic wildness. They may have unwittingly hated their bodies or needed to dissociate from them in order to enjoy pleasure, but they evoked tenderness and affinity in me. This was the greatest pleasure my project gave me: liking people at their worst, in their moments of purgatory.

A Novice's Glossary

Daddy (butch sadist); Boy (butch masochist); lipstick lesbian (a lesbian who dresses by fashionable feminine stereotypes); TB (transbisexual); TS/G (transgendered; same as Gender Variant Folk); metamorph (a person who believes in sustaining physical ambiguity; a gender switch); Goth (a punk who favors heavy makeup and Gothic outfits); boychick (a woman in boys' clothes and haircut); radical fairy (a purposefully effeminate gay man); JAP (Jewish-American princess).

I n the Castro Street dance club a blindfolded girl, hands tied behind her back, bends over the counter of the bar next to a stack of neat white cocktail napkins. The soundtrack plays Roberta Flack, Wishbone, Nina Simone. Young women swing to the music. The girl lying against the counter has short red hair elegantly shaved at the nape, freckled skin, defiantly bulging neck muscles, a tiny mustache. The unapologetic smack of soft black leather against her soft white skin assiduously echoes.

The girl wielding the bullwhip wears a baseball hat backwards over cropped black hair, black latex pants, combat boots. The two girls look alike, but the dominant lacks the wide-eyed, cleansed glow of the submissive. Nearly every woman in attendance has short hair, prominent cheekbones, conspicuous biceps, and thick efficient hands. The air is tense with feral desire. The dominant "tops" carry an undefinable weight that makes their shoulders stoop; a sullen reserve clouds their eyes; this makes it easy to distinguish them from the "bottoms," who display a freshness and an ingenuous joie de vivre one does not expect in women who get off being spanked and flogged and slashed and carved.

This is what "Daddy" is about to do as she swings open a barber's straight razor that looks sharp enough to split hairs. "Are you Daddy's Boy?" she asks the blindfolded redhead, plunging the gleaming edge into the sacrificial nape. "Yes," the prone "Boy" whispers with a sigh of pleasure, "I am your Boy." She keeps utterly still, fervent with the consciousness of being watched. The razor breaks her skin. She bites her lip. Daddy keeps a hand on Boy's nape protectively, and caressingly runs the blade against her back. Blood trickles out. The strokes become shorter and quicker, like accelerating sexual thrusts, until Daddy moans and, dramatically fast, cuts with firm precision small parallel X's from one shoulder to the other. The rest of us watch and sip nonalcoholic drinks as, in a simulation of a postcoital spurt, Daddy gives up all aim and slashes at random. Blood spurts, painting them pagan. "I open you like no fist can open you," Daddy says in a controlled voice. As if that were a cue, the Boy starts to scream for mercy. She sounds impetuous and celebratory. She has crossed over to another side.

San Francisco *is* America's other side. It doesn't try to hide its transgressions in crowds or mansions, in single-family detachable Crestwoods or Dairy Queen parking lots. In San Francisco, sex is not artless; it is accessible but labyrinthine. Bumper stickers read "Sex is the answer. What is the question?" The local papers advertise classes, offered on a sliding scale, in Cupping and Waxing, Caning for Pain, Rape & Terror Fantasy, C&B Torture. The Academy of Body Modification offers instruction in Deprivation, Constriction, Contortion, Distention, where students are suspended from flesh hooks, skewered, or hung. The Institute for the Advanced Study of Human Sexuality has the largest sex library in the world (including the largest collection of porn, housed in eight warehouses), offers a sexual restructuring program called Fuckarama that involves the simultaneous projection of porn films, and awards fully accredited master's degrees in sexology. The natives patronize corsetries, boutiques that sell Würtenburg wheels, Victorian parlors, Edwardian attics, "handballing soirées," "electroplay charity fund-raisings." The streets brim with Gender Variant Folk, Granddaddies and G-spot Mommies, bulldaggers, adult babies, PVC boy-toys and sex-maids, and infinite combinations thereof (top-femme-hookers, butch-bottom-cocksuckers, androgynous leather doggies, radical bi fistfuckers) and somehow all these categories remain distinct and readily understood via clothes and markings and hairdos. San Franciscans take their pleasure meticulously and devoutly. Like its namesake, St. Francis's city doesn't think skin is holy so much as a path to holiness—the spirit's battlefield and playground. Here the human body is a window-shop, a self-avenging tool, a devotional map, a signpost to transcendence.

The town is a constellation of colonies delimited by their esoteric forms of pleasure. Their members identify themselves by acronyms (TV, TB, TS/G, FTM, MTF) and external codes (lipstick lesbian, boychick, tribal, fairy, Goth, metamorph). Issues of trust are paramount in these small communities that feel persecuted by mainstream America, and semantics are disproportionately important as means of recognition in a hostile world—like the Masons' rings and handshakes, or the early Christians' fish acronym* and sign of the cross. These denizens see themselves as sexual outlaws. Rebels with a carnal cause, they employ the classical tactics of insurgents: secrecy, solidarity, insulation. Their sexuality makes them feel communally connected in an increasingly disconnected world. They inadvertently create their own sanctimonious status quo.

*"ΙΧθΥΣ" is an acronym that stands for Jesus Christ Song of God Savior. "ΙΧθΥΣ" means fish as one word.

The S/M lesbians who have rented this club for the night are emblematic of these modern, sexually charged enclaves. In their day lives, they are accountants, florists, cops, day-school teachers. They are friendly, warm, empathic, intellectually lively, and predictable. But at night they are petulant, horny, belligerent, suspicious. Tonight most either ignore me disdainfully or they hawkishly size me up. Have I shed my blood to a woman? Have I been inducted? Have I proven myself? I assume my toughest pose and sip my cranberry juice soberly, hoping to pass for a visiting blood sister.

A new couple has replaced the performers in the corner of the bar. This Daddy is a leather Topman dyke with an unflinching thin-lipped expression and a thigh harness that prominently displays the hunting knife she is carrying. She effortlessly delivers fast, crashing blows with a paddle on her Boy's ass. The blond Boy's face is buried against the counter where the barwoman hands out energy shakes. Most customers watch the archetypal show attentively; a few slowdance or make out on the dance floor.

With one hand Daddy reaches around to tug at Boy's nipple ring, and with the other brushes the Boy's clit, and simultaneously thrusts her silicone strap-on dildo into the Boy's vagina. Daddy pumps the Boy hard, holding her by the hair, panting, groaning, and yelling, then suddenly stops, just short of climaxing, and pulls out. Boy keeps writhing. The smack of Daddy's paddle reprimands her. Boy stops still, trained. Daddy slides her left latex-gloved fist into the Boy's ass. Her right hand unsheathes the knife. "Spill your blood for me, Boy," Daddy commands, her voice thin and sane. Her knife cuts shorter deeper incisions than the razor had earlier. The blade springs blood all over the Boy's plump ass. "I pour my blood for you," Boy vows in an ecstatic loud whisper. Something unspeakable, almost mystical, is taking place here, an evocation of brutal medieval Passion Plays. For two thousand years, Christianity has defined love as submission to an infallible

Daddy; it taught us to obey codes and canons determined by "fathers"; to value the lover who appears invulnerable over an insecure equal. Boys remind me of lambs and Daddies of priests who demand absolute faith to assure their sovereignty. The religiosity of this performance is profoundly shocking. Shredding each thigh in equidistant parallels, Daddy rubs her face in each laceration and laps up the fresh blood. "I give you all of me," Boy mumbles dramatically. "My faith is my blood." Their shadows rage red on the wall as they climax—left fist in ass, dildo in vagina, right hand cutting flesh.

A stocky young brunette in full leather finery and horn-rimmed glasses grasps my shoulder just then and I jolt in irrational panic, scared that her touch has made my blood pour out. Embarrassed by my still bristling body, by the unfailing atavism of instinctive fear, I start to apologize—"Sorry, I'm tense"—when she says, in a scratchy singsong, "Let me inside you." She means under my skin. She shifts her weight open-legged, expectantly, and smiles devilishly: "Are you a virgin?" No, I reply, bewildered, only later realizing I was lying, because she meant virgin to knifeplay. "You don't like to be watched?" she baits me again, in a tone that seems to ask: What's wrong with you? I feel defective, for I'm only the note-taking spectator of noble bloodthirsty warriors, the craven archivist of a breathtaking carnage.

Her name is Electra, she is twenty-six, getting her MBA at Berkeley. She has a baby face and a nasal twang. I buy her a drink at another bar. She tells me she discovered cutting as a teenager in Arizona. One night, feeling dramatic after an adolescent breakup, she jumped off a loading dock; she accidentally landed in a pile of glass. "I had this revelation of my blood: it didn't hurt, it was ecstasy. I went home bleeding and feeling powerful, full of myself. I was over my breakup just like that. But I wanted to have that rush again." After that, she periodically cut herself, she says, "as an exercise in self-restraint and a test of willpower; and out of curiosity about my own limits, like walking barefoot on hot asphalt. Once I slashed each of my fingertips to change my fingerprints." It didn't work.

"My father raised me to think I was better than everyone else, enrolled me in accelerated school programs, spoiled me silly; it took me a long time to quit being a monster and learn about suffering. Suffering," she explains, "is patience. Suffering makes life interesting. When I cut myself, I'm not suicidal. I'm too much in control for that. I am *alive:* blood is a reaffirmation of life. Because of another part of my sexual history—I was sexualized by my brother, the normal American story—I had a leg up on my anorexic girlfriends. I was more mature, and I was a great liar. I could manipulate people too easily; but when I slivered off my skin and saw my insides, I felt real. Violence is the ultimate reality." She grinds her teeth, looking so well-scrubbed, gentle, and huggable that I'm not convinced of her proclaimed malevolence. Can fury smell so clean? "I constantly want to kill people," she insists. "I'm not opposed to violence." I think she just doesn't want to be rapable.

The last time she cut herself she was in a lecture hall, right after the breakup of another longtime relationship. She realized she had been dragging her keys across the side of her wrist when the person next to her yelled, "You're bleeding." The school called an ambulance. "I was just having a private moment," she complains, "but it turned into a public spectacle. I'd lost control of myself." She stopped cutting herself after that. For the next five years she only cut her lovers exclusively for sex. But last week she bought a new "butterfly knife" and, walking home drunk with it, had the urge to try it out. She came home bleeding. Her girlfriend, Esther, thought she had been mugged. It was cathartic, but Electra now wishes she hadn't given in to impulse; she likes to keep her cutting within the safe parameters of mutual erotic pleasure. She shows me her scars from that last incident: three thick white lines that sunburst out of her wrist like exclamation points. They disappear into a tattoo of a hunting knife that covers her bulky forearm. She also has tattoos of *Hello Kitty*, a few gargoyles, medieval alchemy symbols, a knife-pierced heart that reads "Esther," and the Chinese characters for "PAIN" on her other forearm. "They're my talismans," she explains, resorting to biblical language. In a perverse way, she's turned her body into a church. Her goal is panhistoric and simple: keep evil out. "My tattoos relate a coherent, thought-out story, but they don't weigh as much as my scars in terms of documents. I like to document my life, to own it. Every scar tells a story—a war story."

Now she only cuts Esther. "I love to ingest her blood; it sounds cliché, but it's really ingesting someone's essence, going inside her and not killing her, which is the epitome of power. It's true possession of my lover, marking territory. It's a complete connection, because at the most profound level my lover's life is in my hands. And it is emotionally sexy that someone accepts and loves me even though I put the knife to her, and trusts me with it. It's total love, surrender. Esther's skin is my canvas." She tells me she yearns for a more authoritarian, comforting, settled society. It's the familiar allure of religion. Theologically speaking, her lover's blood rises from the sea of her yearning.

The first person Electra cut beside herself was a lover during a monumental fight they had over an infidelity. She held an antique military knife to her lover's neck and called her a bitch. "I cut her only because she moved. It was a fluke, but I couldn't believe how erotic it felt. We didn't talk about it. It was frightening for both of us. It was a leap of faith. It tore up the affair. She couldn't handle it. I, too, get overwhelmed sometimes and get flashes of revulsion. I mean, it *is* human blood."

At the end of the night, Electra takes me home to introduce

me to her "bottom," Esther. Their apartment is cathedral-ceilinged and dorm room–like, littered with inch-deep dirt, ashes, and dog hair. Heaps of clothes, books, notes, decaying snacks, and found objects are strewn about. Esther is a pretty black-haired JAP, an honors classics student in sixties tight polyester hiphuggers, short blue nails, and dark red lipstick. She has a feline allure and a comical sorority-girl accent, and speaks in quick fluid bursts, as if she must hurry and express each thought before she changes her mind. There is a studied jadedness and a cool anger in her deep-set eyes. She seems unusually smart.

"When we do it, Electra gets my blood all over her face and looks like a complete savage," Esther chuckles merrily, sitting on Electra's pudgy lap. "Blood is such an aphrodisiac; it takes us to totally heightened orgasms—female orgasms. The secret is that we never start with cutting, or cut to punish. We warm up to it, we kiss and she whips me to bring my blood to the surface; and I drink red wine first so my blood won't coagulate as fast. We do cutting on special occasions, like smoking a cigar. To celebrate. Blood is a dangerous sport these days, but we're both tested and we're strictly monogamous. I'd like to try it in public, but we're not part of the community. We're trying to break in." She seems to be speaking to the city more than to me.

Esther bears a tattoo of Electra's name in a knife-pierced heart on her breast, and chunky metal studs through her tongue, eyebrow, chin, navel, and nipples. Her smooth white shoulders are crisscrossed by faint whiter scars from sexual cuts, of the messy type pro cutters call hamburger cuts. It might offend her to have her scars called delicate, but they are: pale skin doesn't scar deeply. I have to peer close to detect Esther's gentle documents of lust. "Love is way overrated," she chortles. "People are always ready to deliberate the morality of violence and some similar timeless question, but to me it's basic life stuff: Electra is my family. I chose her. Our sex feels great. End of story." I realize a scar signifies a forced ending, a closure, conclusion, completion, which is the teleological goal of every ritual sacrifice: divine perfection.

Esther tells me her father, a famous Fort Lauderdale plastic surgeon, is horrified by her piercings, yet he himself has had a nose job and has resculpted his new wife. "He wants to do my nose, but I won't let him. I tell him if he wants to make my nose smaller, it's out of penis envy. It makes him squirm. His surgery is like our cutting," she giggles. "Every day Dad cuts scars into women's faces and breasts that take six months, not two weeks, to heal. Half of those women get crushes on him and keep going back. They can never get enough; he's like a guru to them. They depend on him more than I do on Electra. But *that's* not taboo, because stapling their bellies makes them into better erotic objects for men. Well, my difference is I do it with my eyes open, I don't use anesthetics. I'm honest. I do it for the experience." Socially sanctioned surgical cutting is a sign of affluence and success in an America that continues to prize Aryan homogeneity. Women enjoy not the act of it but the resulting scar. *That* scar is associated with an illusion of youth, an erasure of life's marks, an undocument. For some it's a symbolic rebirth, a second chance. But for lesbians like Esther it is conveyor-belt remodeling that steals away a woman's soul. And though they don't mention this connection, I now wonder if they incorporate scalpels and cuts into their sex lives as a reaction to the "violence" of our cosmetic correction system.

Kim is an alabaster-beautiful, mellow twenty-four-year-old Korean I strike up a conversation with at The Bearded Lady café. She is the adopted daughter of white Christian intellectuals. She publishes a "grrl" 'zine and studies design at the Art Institute. She's soon telling me she first cut circles into her belly while tripping on mushrooms and black gels. "I did it because bodies are so plain. People make too big a deal out of them. We're too caught up in the physical world, in money and sex; we have problems because we put so much emphasis on all *that*. People don't see the body for what it is, just a space to hold our spirit, like a shell; so they think blood is scary. People judge you by your body, though when you're born you don't have a choice, it's got nothing to do with *you*. I'm sick of being told I'm pretty. My looks don't let me get close to people. It's like a screen. So I do my scars, to remind myself of my own core, and to scare people off and show I'm tougher than I look, especially because I am small. I defy them. I know it won't kill me. Blood is familiar, close. I scar out of boredom, to keep occupied, or to feel involved in something real. It's like, 'Yeah! I did it!' It's like an accomplishment—the one thing I can always feel successful about. Sometimes life feels pointless, full of people coming and going, and that's a good time to make a cut, a mark on yourself, like a reminder. I like to carry my history written on my flesh." Self-inflicted violence seems to be the main prop of her self-respect.

Women like Kim draw blood in what resembles a decorous masturbation, in an effort to discover a more authentic part of themselves, unaffected by outside designations and disguises. They feel so alien from the bodies they possess that touching is not enough to convince them that they are real. It's not the female lack of penis, or the lack of danger invoked by the difference between male and female size and strength, that has introduced violence into lesbian sex. The body is our first means of organizing our experience; the mind, being forever manipulable, complicates life. Pain is simple. Blood reassures them by evoking a time-honored reality: inside our bodies, we're all the same. Fragility facilitates intimacy. Blood also achieves an equilibrium between the realm of artifice in which we function and the biological reality we inhabit. Bloodshed disturbs the somnolent order of things. A wound reminds us that we exist.

Hester is another young lesbian whose history is exorcised on her flesh. She is an incest survivor, though she is loath to associate that with her cutting. She paints murals at banks and teaches art in a vocational school. She is rosy-cheeked and sparkling clean in her khaki overalls and lace undershirt. She speaks in a soothing benevolent voice, enunciating meticulously as if carefully removing each word from its wrappings. Because she is strong and stubborn in daily life, she says, she likes to be submissive in sex; doing things she may not want to do turns her on. "It's hard to admit it publicly," she explains, sitting politely in my hotel room. "Women have spent so much time earning respect and claiming their independence; but it's peaceful not to have to be in control for a while. Love between women is outside the rules anyway."

Hester grew up in Shaker Heights, the daughter of a celebrated civic leader who joined the Rajneesh cult and left the family. She's had panic attacks and body memories, but no conscious memories, of incestual abuse. "My S/M violation claims that old icky violation back, because it's conscious, consensual, and clearly delineated. I *own* my body now. I *use* my scars to remember." She has the loveliest scar I've seen: a 3-D skin sculpture, a spiral of overlapping flesh petals rising out of the center of her sternum like a pink bud. "I thought about this for three years before I got it," she says. "To me, cutting and scarification are different. I do not cut myself thoughtlessly, because it can imply self-hatred. But self-scarification is an anchor, a return to my body, a lasting conversation with my body as I take care of it while it heals. I got this scar when my mother died; I went through a cycle of depression and when I came out of it I wanted a spiral on my grief spot. My lover, who is a nurse, cut it with a scalpel. It hurt less than a paper cut. We made a ritual out of it: my friends held me as she did it. We burned incense, read invocations. We've done more since then, one on our bellies that we cut on each other, and a recent one of a phoenix made of runes that she cut on me at a public sex party. This was our coming out as cutters. I only let my lover cut me, because cutting is a psychic orgasm. It creates incredible intimacy. All my scars are my emotional centers, signs of a life lived."

I had met with a lot of reticence and mistrust from the cutters I'd tried to contact. But Hester and her lover were visible in the community and her visit gave me a seal of approval. That very evening their friend Molly, a twenty-seven-year-old assistant director of photography with a tense seriousness occasionally interrupted by a big goofy smile, took me to the Eros club for a women's S/M night.

The club provides S/M playrooms, a maze of curtained-off hospital-like beds, showers, saunas, a video lounge. Molly comes here for safe blood play. "It's like going to the gym for me," she says in her breathy high voice. "Afterwards I feel lighter and energized." She was first sexually cut at eighteen. "We'd walk down the street and my girlfriend would pull a knife on me under my sweater and say, 'Keep moving,' like in a stickup. I'd feel all my fears gather up on the surface where I had to confront them; but I was in the safest place in the world, in my lover's arms, so my mind could let go of fear. She cut me and then fucked my brains out. I've been into it ever since. I don't really enjoy sex without it. Too tame."

At the foyer we sign release forms and pick up gloves, dental dams, and condoms. The first sight I encounter is that of a thin girl in a leather Merry Widow with long needles piercing her mouth and cheeks. I join the small crowd in disbelief. There is no ecstasy here. A mirthless dyke in jeans is coolly inserting hypodermic needles in and out of the girl's flesh. Every time her skin pops, a lot of blood trickles down her pallid face. It is a gut-wrenching spectacle. Molly tells me it hurts more to watch than to do. She's had it done, and it's not a high except for exhibitionists who get off on the attention the amount of blood generated draws. "When the needle goes into the muscle, you feel a dull static buzz under your skin, nothing compared to the sharp sting of a razor." She laughs it off and turns to watch an old-fashioned feather-boa striptease in an adjacent room. I can't avert my eyes from the martyr.

"Play-piercing requires technique," the piercer tells me when she is done. "I'm a perfectionist; I like to space needles even and pretty; I lace them up in figure-eight loops; then I pull the threads. *That* feels real good to her. Like with any breaking of skin, the endorphins kick in very fast, and that's what makes blood sports better than other S/M trips. These are spinal tap needles. For the bottom, it's a sensational endurance test. For a top, it's pride in years of study and hard work."

Molly has run into her friend Liz, who happens to be blind-folded and tied by her dog collar to a side table. Liz vigorously extends her hand in my aural direction and says, smiling and shaking mine, "Tell me what you want." She's waiting for her lover, a dentist and "classic Daddy," who is doing another scene. "Being Daddy's Boy is a safe way for me to be nurtured," she immediately explains in what seems to me a self-conscious euphoria. I feel as if I have fallen in with a league of amateur ideological commissars that bring to my mind Mao's child-sol-diers of the Cultural Revolution. Is the sanctity of the body defunct? "I feel too vulnerable as a girl—anything approaching a wife is way too scary. I was raised a tomboy. But, with all the cutting I do, the only permanent scars I have are from throat surgery." I decide to lift her blindfold. She humors me.

She's a New Englander who moved to San Francisco, after graduating from Radcliffe, to "get away from the antiporn les-bian feminists who think S/M is violence against women that perpetuates the oppression of patriarchy, that it's women tak-ing on the bad habits of men. Those bitches are frigid. It's Salem territory out there." She's an engaging thirty-three-year-old with sandy close-cropped hair, hazel eyes, a broad smile. Her sensible, even tone renders the incongruity of her S/M accouterments progressively invisible, and absurd. "I get off being bitten," she says, wetting her lips, relishing my interest. "I love it when my lover swoops down on me like a vampire and bites me to suck my blood. The sensation of her sucking my blood is incredible, a great sense of peace. All my energy focuses on that spot. After I'm aroused, she slashes me and sucks it all off, or she'll just let it bleed and clot, and I have blood streaks on my body and go to sleep like that. It *looks* fabulous! We've never had to bandage anything. I only use a bandage after I feed my pet leech on my arm."

So is this what women do among themselves when society is not policing? I ask. "It's great feeling primal," Molly confirms as we continue our Dantean stroll. We mill around. Girls are kicked and mauled in dim corners. We briefly pause before a nymphet in lingerie who looks like a Victoria's Secret model, hanging from a ceiling hook. Her friends, all young and elated, urge us to whip her; they behave both like cheerleaders and spiritual advisers. It is her birthday, they say, and they had promised her "the classic" one hundred smacks. Molly offers to use her knife. The girl squeals, I believe happily.

We move on, exchanging greetings with naked, half-naked, and elaborately dressed women of every size and hue. Some carry floggers draped over their shoulders or bagfuls of clothespins and clips. In the darkest rooms, parallel rows of curtained beds host less flashy, more sincere sex. All the beds are occupied. A long line of hugging, kissing, groaning girls forms outside, waiting to use them. I have the feeling that a clandestine collective civil experiment is being conducted here. I think of W. H. Auden's line, "If we [men] ever discovered what women say to each other when we are not there, our male vanity might receive such a shock that the human race would die out."

"I love blood. It drives me mad," announces a shrill voice ahead. "We dedicate this to Kali." The speaker looks like an eighteen-year-old grunge groupie in striped pants and platform sneakers. Molly says it's a "bloodbath scene." The three girls nod to each other fiercely and simultaneously stick three open-topped twenty-gauge needles in their veins. Blood fountains out. They sing off-key and wail and fingerpaint the walls with it. They put bloody palm prints and lunar-shaped graffiti on each other. A naked girl in a straitjacket and a leather hood stands still nearby, as part of the performance. I am unnerved. It's not much blood, maybe 30 cc out of each arm, much less than the pint people donate at the hospital, but it is uncontained and it has colored everything within reach.

Bloodletting has a canonical past. The many generations who used it as general medicine knew that shedding blood releases tension. Women were the primary beneficiaries of this practice, perhaps because they're more at ease with losing blood and enduring pain. Compared to the menstrual blood shed monthly, the quantities of blood produced by even the most compulsive cutting are negligible. Compared to birth pains, the sting of a blade is innocuous. On the other hand, men generally have a distaste for blood, perhaps because theirs is the hemophiliac gender. The burliest leathermen, I am told, recoil from blood sports; and cutting occurs in straight S/M only if the woman is the cuttee.

In a recent series of brain-stimulation studies, Dr. Paul MacLean (head of the Lab of Brain Evolution and Behavior at the National Institute of Mental Health) identified a neurological link between sex and aggression; he found that the electrical stimulation of a one-millimeter area of the brain, the amygdala, evokes responses of salivation, teeth grinding, fearful or angry vocalizations, and erections. The proximity of the neural structures governing violence and sexual stimulation explains everyday occurrences such as erection after REM sleep or after a domestic fight or an attack. Hostility generates and enhances sexual excitement. Terror, inherent in the struggle for dominance, is erotic. This is one reason why people associate danger with sex. It can also explain blood sports.

Sexual bloodletting is still a minority taste. But scarification as an aesthetic statement is an ancient rite that is making a big culture-wide comeback. When life seems impenetrable or pretentious, when its mysteries are constantly explicated and yet remain unknowable, the body becomes the last bastion for "authentic" self-expression. Scarification has been rediscovered as a tool for actualizing emotions that can't be commonly expressed. Women in particular use scars to defy a society that commodifies looking sexy rather than being sexual. The young crowds at the local Body Manipulations or Nomad or Gauntlet piercing salons clamoring to get their frenums and clit hoods and Prince Alberts and septums and foreskins pierced, giggling and holding hands like live Benetton ads, are products of a society where 90 percent of young white women, according to a *Newsweek*-reported poll, hate their bodies.

But fashion has already made their quest for individuality meaningless. "Piercing is like toothbrushing by now," a male piercer at Nomad informs me. "It's like taking your car in for a paint job." He is covered in solid black "tribal" tattoos that leave only his fingers, face, and toes flesh-toned. His dilated nostrils and earlobes bear bones and bronze bars, but he still looks like a scraggly nerd hiding his neuroses under the mystique of an African male. "It's why cutting is becoming popular," he explains. The professionals at Nomad do cuttings with the tip of a heated cauterizing knife. For lasting scars they recommend branding, using galvanized sheet metal. They are opposed to the use of scalpels, which are "invasive modern Western instruments." At Body Manipulations, on the other hand, the all-women employees cut with scalpels and rub sage ash in the wounds in an Native American tradition to help them scar. These arcane differences may seem humorous, but in the business of nostalgia they translate into profit or loss. Cutters must inspire trust like priests.

Raelyn Gallina, an S/M lesbian, is the best-known professional cutter in San Francisco. For about $60 an hour, she has performed hundreds of cuttings in the past ten years. Celtic knots, tarot cards, or totem animals are the most popular. The designs are chosen by the clients, often from a portfolio of her work composed of actual bloodprints. She rubs tattoo ink in them to ensure permanence, or cuts out wedges to create thicker scar tissue, so the scars won't disappear if the skin is not rich enough in melanin to "keloid." Raelyn says people want cuts "for adornment, or as a warrior's test, or to claim their sexuality, or as a sacrifice that marks an upcoming transformation." Cutting is a difficult craft because of its unpredictability. "Each body scars differently. It's the most natural art, because the body itself creates its scar. It's my job," she adds, "but I do it because I like blood."

So do Claudia and her boyfriend, Blue, two "vampires" known in San Francisco for their blood-drinking performances. In my hotel room, Claudia wolfs down nuts, chocolates, martinis, cigarettes, and the conversation with equal compulsion. She burps, coughs, sweats, and punctually staggers to the bathroom. She has a broken exhausted voice, long dark stringy hair, a tall toneless body, and a breath that wheezes clamorously like an allergy-prone Nosferatu. She is alternately inert and hyper, desperate and confident, seasoned and childish. Her veins are bruised. Her rapid-fire speech is intermittently erudite. At twenty-eight she is a published poet who makes a living as a "vampire stripper" at a strip club by thrusting her hairless labia into the face of any man with close proximity to the stage and grinding her fangs to a bloodcurdling soundtrack and a video of *The Lost Children*.

Blue is a quiet, composed, hyperaware pothead. He has a vulnerable-boy pretty face, a no-nonsense manner, and a guttural grandfatherly voice. He takes his licensed phlebotomist's skills seriously: he and Claudia get paid by clubs to perform "necroporn"—to draw and drink each other's blood and then invite members of the audience to taste their own. If there is a shortage of gigs, Blue, an androgynous twenty-two-year-old, places ads in the paper and finds businessmen willing to pay him $200 to pee on them. He pompously explains, "We believe in alternate ways of making money. Claudia does out-call dominating as a vampire mistress. Lightweight prostitution is like working at McDonald's." "It's my NEA grant," Claudia shouts. "It's easy," Blue adds in his permanently scornful tone, "because people are into young-body worship—and I get a power rush being paid for being young. My body is just a costume for me. Fucking or sticking my tongue in a mouth is part of the disguise. I'm interested in the insides of the body. Getting the blood out is the most personal way to have sex. The other sex we'll do only for money. That's our ethic." Blue is also on welfare and trying to get SSI disability status by convincing the state he is socially dysfunctional because of his vampirism.

The bloodsipping I watch them indulge in is disquieting mostly because it looks mercenary. My body feels overwrought and drained as I watch, like a boxer's as he retires from the ring. There is decadence in their half-naked bodies smeared in blood, but their faces stay businesslike. They are postmodern hawkers of their blood. They display no palpable abandon to justify the bloodsucking climax. The procedure is medical: a twenty-eight-gauge insulin syringe expertly pierces a vein. Once the syringe is full, they shoot the blood into each other's gaping mouths. They swallow, smack their lips, shoot blood on their bodies, and lick it like cum in the way of porn stars. They cavort and grind and caress provocatively but not intimately. Their technique reminds me of late-night phone-sex TV ads. They do not thrill; they trade in our fear of mortality. Their goal is materialistic: to make a living off our nightmares, like they've seen politicians, religious leaders, warmongers, publicists do.

What I find most interesting about Claudia and Blue are their personal histories, because they are common to their generation. Granted, the two spent Valentine's Day at the orthodontist's getting permanent fangs. They sleep in a cus-tom-made double coffin. They are vampire junkies, meaning they shoot heroin to slow down their metabolism and delay old age. They keep out of the sun, take "miracle vitamins" and DHEA hormones, and practice Anton LaVey's postmodern Satanism. ("We're Luciferians, not Church of Satan," Claudia clarifies. "It's the opposite of the AA philosophy.") And every so often they interrupt our chat to ask if I'm sure I don't want to taste my blood, which they could draw here in the hotel room. "I've tasted it," I say. "I suck my finger cuts. It's sticky." "Coppery," Claudia corrects me nonchalantly. "Like sucking on a quarter, but sweeter," Blue sternly adds. But they do it all as if it were a fantasy game ("We're *Nightmare Before Christmas* figures," Blue says. "I'm TankGirlish; in our love, we're Anne Rice characters"), and they are making an American success story out of it. They're local media celebrities. They're New Agers terrified of old age. They are culture victims determined to become cultural paragons. That's why they go out in costume and drag fifteen-year-olds into bathrooms of clubs and order them to blow each other. Unwittingly making this point clear, Blue tells me the biggest vampire in the world must be Michael Jackson: "Note his pale skin, his oxygen tank, his Neverland ranch, his power play with boys. Michael sucks those boys' blood in his own postmodern way."

Claudia's father is a prominent economist who taught at Johns Hopkins, in a city where she was exposed to "a lot of scary Catholic iconography at school." She always wanted to stand out; so her first Hollywood Dracula movie showed her a way out of a boring uneventful life. Blue was raised in the Virgin Islands' sunshine by doting working-class parents who fattened him up. He grew to hate daylight and sports. In his teens, he legally changed his Christian name and set out to create an original identity. Both suffered the typical adolescent alienation of suburban life in the eighties and starred in their own pop myths in order to escape a narrow reality, as most creatively inclined kids do. Media-educated and lonesome, they identified with the power and loneliness of vampires.

One day little Claudia pricked herself, tasted her blood, and liked the forbidden sensation; another day she spooned out her menstrual blood, tasted it, and felt empowered by her transgression. So she dressed as a witch and cut herself once a month, alone in her room at a makeshift altar. When she and Blue met, they found in each other a mirror image that inspired them. They went through a period of sexual exploration, tried phlebotomy in a friend's dungeon, and found that they "enjoyed doing this more than anything else in the world." And with this they also found their identities.

"Middle class order is only disorder," wrote René Magritte. "Disorder to the point of paroxysm, deprived of all contact with the world of necessity." Middle-class America motivates the nonsexual bloodletting that is now prevalent among teens and was the starting point for many sexual cutters. Adolescents carve words, pictures, and haphazard slashes into their arms, legs, chest, stomach, face, or genitals. They use knives, paper clips, needles, scissors, tacks, pieces of glass, or even fingernails. They cut to get attention, or to experience a pseudosuicide, or to substitute physical pain for an overwhelming nebulous inner pain they can't name or control. They say they cut to let out "demons and poisons," unknowingly emulating initiation rites and superstitions as old as the Stone Age. They pack a razor to school or to Grandma's for a quick fix of pain "to get through the day," because as soon as a cut unleashes blood, they feel "a rush of relief, like popping the lid off a pressure cooker," and also a sensation of control and fearlessness. They don't cut to die, but the reverse: they hurt themselves "to feel something; to feel alive," they say, "to feel better." It's a shocking repudiation of our common sense.

Different psychiatrists have called this overwhelming compulsion to break skin "a partial suicide to avoid a total suicide," "a desire not to die, but to feel something," "a way of self-soothing," "a coping mechanism," "an act of self-help";

they have associated it with a range of psychiatric problems, including depression, obsessive-compulsive disorder, multiple or borderline personality disorder, and most often with childhood traumas such as physical or sexual abuse, loss, abandonment, neglect, illness, or injury. In a six-month study at the UCSF inpatient psychiatric unit in 1988, 83 percent of those who reported sexual abuse engaged in cutting, presumably in self-punishment (it is the fault of the body that it can get hurt or abused by another's desire, the reasoning goes; if one is invulnerable to physical pain and danger, one is free).

"A cut is very ordinary," Molly told me. "You chop vegetables and cut yourself. You shave your legs and cut yourself. You break a glass and cut yourself. People do it all the time. It's no worse if you do it on purpose, except it's easier because you're prepared for it. You let go, and you cut." As a kid, whenever she was angry or stressed, she'd press her brother's Swiss Army knife against her thumb and watch it slowly break skin. "It brought my every molecule into focus for a moment. And I'd go, 'Aaah, I feel better now.' My brother punched walls instead. But, as with everything, if you're compulsive about it and develop a daily habit, it becomes a disorder; people who use it to escape reality become fanatics and are dependent on it. It can be a double-edged sword. No pun."

"Self-mutilation is the exact opposite of suicide," claims Armando Favazza, a professor of psychiatry at the University of Missouri, in the October 1997 issue of *I-D*. "People who mutilate themselves want to feel better." There are no statistics about the numbers of sexual cutters, but the literature on compulsive self-cutting is substantial. An estimated 2 million Americans currently engage in self-cutting. Favazza, author of the book *Bodies Under Siege* and coauthor of the largest study ever of self-mutilators, estimates that 750 out of every 100,000 Americans have deliberately harmed themselves at some point. Addicts range from preteens to eighty-year-old housewives. But the typical chronic self-mutilator, he says, is a white woman in her midtwenties to early thirties, middle or upper-middle class, intelligent, and successful, who began injuring herself at around age fourteen and has injured herself at least fifty times.

The practice has long been common in gangs and prisons. But the more general addiction is a recent and fast-spreading phenomenon. The newsletter *Cutting Edge,* Self-Mutilators Anonymous (SMA), and a program called SAFE (Self-Abuse Finally Ends) all offer support for those "living with SIV (self-inflicted violence)." Abstinence is the only official prescription for recovery (although many people like Electra find that sexualizing their cutting helps them control it). "Pathological cutting," as therapists call it, remains largely untreated because most cutters never "come out." The first inpatient treatment program for self-mutilators opened in Chicago's Hartgrove Hospital only in 1985. SIV still carries the stigma that drug addiction, alcoholism, or anorexia used to. It is seen as an "unnatural act," a morbid regression to unevolved tribal customs. Even though the practice is less debilitating or habit-forming than most compulsions, it remains taboo. Yet because self-cutting is done in isolation and people rarely share cutting tools, it carries negligible HIV risk. Physically, it is no more damaging than hiking through the woods and getting scratched by thorns. Intellectually, it is no more harmful, in my estimation, than a daily dose of "90210." And for those who wear their scars as "badges of honor," it may not be physically damaging either. What I do find disquieting is that its scars are advertisements for the invisible scars of an increasingly violent and hollow society. By its extreme cry for attention, cutting proves how difficult everyday communication has become; it reveals the dormant hunger for passion, individual expression, and meaningful contact that stirs under our cloistered, cyberized, smoke-screened world. In this, the century of Bergen-Belsen and Dachau and the Khmer Rouge, it turns out that Stephen Dedalus (James Joyce's alter ego) was wrong: history is not the nightmare from which we are all trying to awake, but the nightmare we are trying to re-create—in a last-ditch attempt to wrench awake the safely narcotized confines of our homes.

We live in a blood-drenched society: much of our daily entertainment consists of reenactments of manslaughter in movies, books, news stories, the arts; our medicine, our sense of valor, our national history, our very birth, are steeped in blood. Many of us derive our spiritual sustenance from the communal partaking of the blood of the son of God. Many of us, in the appropriate context, consider bloodshed a romantic act. It's no surprise our sexual imagination can also be blood-driven. Sex predates our reasoning and may always, and possibly for the best, stay inaccessible to it. This is what I am thinking as I mingle with the women who engage in blood sports. I don't find them revolting because I recognize the ancestral apocalyptic metaphors that compel them and I feel that, very deeply and disturbingly, we may all share this barbaric impulse. After all, Jesus' undying power is in his hallow, self-inflicted wounds.

Dallas:
The Economy of Desire

"What is the fleshy part around the vagina called?—
Woman."

Customer at a strip club

An editor called from Spin *with the idea to have me investigate
the working life of a famous strip club (Hollywood was in the
midst of releasing a slew of films on the topic). Because I had
been neglecting my obligations as a magazine staff writer, I
undertook this project even though the subject seemed to me
quite stale. I made dutiful rounds of strip clubs night after
night, talking to the inmates, and saw hundreds of female genitals until I couldn't behold them lucidly any longer. I felt like
Picasso at the beginning of his cubist period.*

*It was at that time I first noticed that my research had con-
sistently revolved around walled-off clubs rather than spontaneous happenings. We now flirted in restricted areas—bars,
clubs, parties—at designated times: after dark. Under the pretense that we respond to each other's minds independently of
each other's bodies, and that, on the other extreme, what we sexually desire in each other is the body alone, we've organized our
civic life around inflexible parameters for acceptable natural
behavior, and defiled our fundamental freedoms.*

Sexual harassment cases broke out in the news every day

and I couldn't but notice the connection. It seemed that a work-ingman couldn't make a pass without running the risk of finding himself in a court of law and losing everything—respect, money, family, job. The day loomed near when a man who asked a woman at a cocktail party to go home with him would face an undercover cop reading him his "rights." This struck me as the revival of the misogynist honor code that had once pitted brother and father of the coveted woman against the brave lover who made a verbal pass at her, which, if the suitor was deemed socially unsuitable or was unwilling to proceed to marriage, gave the family males the right to see to moral justice, often with their guns. The assumption had been that the female in question was a familial property to be bartered, and that female sexuality should be incapable of initiative. (My own father had spent his youth hiding from relatives of girls he had dishonored by simply desiring them.) Now a federal law had reestablished that dialectic: being rejected by an available woman was crimi-nal harassment, being accepted was love, and courting a legally unavailable woman was sheer villainy. In the face of this, many adults shirked all impromptu mating games and found refuge in the safe boundaries of designated sex clubs. Ergo, the resurging popularity of strip clubs.

What has been blurring the difference between consensual fun and harassment is the new idea that sex in any unequal power relation entails coercion. But as I discovered again and again, the relations between lovers, just as between friends, rel-atives, or colleagues, are always, and unavoidably, unequal, mutable, and implosive.

As I first go into a "premier men's club," my body tingles at the abrupt exposure to the bodily secrets of a hun-dred female strangers. For several minutes I experi-ence a peeping-Tom cornucopia, searching every nook with a rush of transgression. Then, much too soon, the glut becomes trite and the artificiality glaring. So when a giantess bends into my face, canines gleaming, goods ingeniously arranged on five-inch spikes and sprinkled with silver glitter, and asks with an aggressive amiability if I'd like a lap dance, I no longer tingle. Her bloated nipples stroke my nose. In extreme close-up the lipstick on her iconic lascivious smile bleeds. But to reward her gender-blindness, I shell out a crisp $20.

"I like showing off to women," she says, while shedding her Lycra, cupping her mammoth breasts, and fingering her nipples, "but the only women clients are Mafiosi molls or ugly wives of meek guys; none of them buy. Are you gay? I only date women—keeps my private and work lives separate." Skimming her waist inches from my clenched lips, she adds: "Eighty-five percent of strippers are gay." I can't see past the vacancy in her eyes.

"It hurts shaking my tits," she goes on good-naturedly, shaking them nonetheless. "But tits are money. If you can carry them as big as your skin will stretch, you hit the jackpot just taking Polaroids with tourists. If you push thirty, you need double Ds to compete." She prattles with the hyperbolic geniality of salespeople. But the unsettling incongruity between her actions and her speech makes it hard to understand the simplest things she says. I say I'm astonished at her unapologetic frankness. "I lie to those who pay me to lie," she replies, twirling her arms to and fro, planting her heel by my crotch, her leg arched, her eyes hawkishly scouting my black-tied neighbors. "The only thoughts that give me comfort at work are castration fantasies. I run slide projections in my head of slicing penises like vegetables." When the song is over, she gives me the customary peck on the cheek and tiptoes off, her face set in a cordial mask. I watch her puppeteer her body toward the next table and realize a stripper is cartoonishly two-dimensional, like a dollar bill. It seems a fair exchange.

Most consumers around me are beefy, short-haired men

with uniformly rigid bodies and stoic, craggy faces—men of fortitude who mind their own business and are alive only to practical purposes. They now act as platoon soldiers on leave. We are in a specially designated space reserved for the discharge of psychic pollution; these men visit it periodically to be emptied of unfit and superfluous desires and then resume their familial and professional slots reliably "clean." The purpose of the modern gentleman's club is less erotic than cathartic.

The strip industry underwent a colossal revolution in the eighties, when super clubs (the sex industry's equivalent of Wendy's and the Gap) came on the scene to service an emerging class of overpaid young professionals, just as AIDS was injecting the element of fear into casual sex. Michael J. Peters, the federally convicted owner of the MJP Dollhouses of America chain, is credited with opening the first super club in Florida in 1982. According to *U.S. News & World Report*, the number of strip clubs has roughly doubled since 1987, and Americans now spend more money at these clubs than they do at the theater, the opera, the ballet, and jazz and classical music concerts combined. Academics hold conferences on the meaning of striptease, and former strippers write tell-all tomes. By 1997, the monotonously titillating overexposure of the subject in the media (with the hyped celluloid version of Carl Hiaasen's book *Striptease* released on the heels of *Showgirls* and *Exotica*) has made strippers into household images. The jiggling of naked nameless flesh has been sanitized. Red-light districts have become X-rated theme parks replete with Broadway-style sets, sunken pits, and vapor pouring out of chrome vents. This legitimization of a pastime that typically needs to be ill-lit to be exhilarating encapsulates America's core genius: its adeptness at dynamically exploiting human instincts for profit while deflating any potentially rebellious impious movements by mass-marketing them into fads.

Of course, these Las Vegas–style gentlemen's clubs are only the latest link in an age-old tradition that includes the harems of the Moguls and the Ottomans, the hetaerae of classical Greece, the temple whores of ancient Egypt, the geishas of Japan. Most of those early upscale adult entertainers were prized not only for their beauty and erotic arts but also for their encyclopedic literary, musical, and conversational skills, their intellectuality and argumentativeness and accumulated wisdom. The modern emancipation of women has made male access to the female mind easily available and even unavoidable, while it has complicated unrestrained male access to girlie flesh. What today's men value the most in a strip bar is their freedom from the dangers and anxieties of the politically correct mating game. Good strippers have no opinions.

"*Cabaret Royale:* Explore the Fantasy," read the ubiquitous flyers in my hotel lobby. In 1988 an innovative Lebanese entrepreneur threw massive capital into a single luxury strip club, applying the fantasy-selling tricks of Hollywood. The result was featured in "Lifestyles of the Rich and Famous," *Playboy, Details, Vogue, Allure*. And because of its size and visibility, its pioneering unabashed advertising, and its unprecedented success, the government chose Cabaret Royale to be one of its two landmark cases in 1995 that led to the closing and reorganizing of every "super" strip club.

By the end of the eighties the gentlemen's clubs' tremendous growth had drawn IRS attention. Until then, strippers were independent contractors who paid clubs stage rent, earned tax-free cash, and chose their own schedules, music, costumes. In 1989, the Department of Labor's Wage and Hour Division organized the GCSF (Gentlemen's Club Strike Force) to enforce a classification of strippers as employees. This ruling enabled the IRS to hold clubs responsible for accumulated Social Security levies, penalizing them heavily and sending most into bankruptcy. The courts upheld the rule, even though the clubs had been a legally vested business and spent millions in legal fees. In the landmark Cabaret case, the courts decided that table-dance tips were club fees to employees for their services; and the Cabaret was fined $11 million in back-wage liabilities. The government wanted in on the action.

Cabaret went bankrupt, changed owners, and now uses the clients' tips to meet the dancers' minimum wage requirements. Bouncers keep track of how much a dancer earns on the floor. If she makes less than minimum wage, the club pays her the difference (or fires her). Dancers declare their cash (though rarely more than the minimum), file income tax and deductions; at the end of each shift, they stop by the "cage," a dingy basement booth manned by a chubby female accountant, and clock out.

IRS spies are the main reason men's clubs are weary of journalists. "When you start digging, who knows what you'll fish out. The adult industry is a closed shop—a private club," publicity managers of the most famous strip clubs repeatedly told me. My quest ends at Cabaret Royale, which bids me welcome only because it is eager to show the public its new clean face. Even so, as Nina, its overworked PR coordinator, picked me up at the Dallas airport in her red sports car, she seemed nervous about our arrangement. She handed me a "schedule": I was allotted two days in the club, under her supervision.

Cabaret is Texas-big. It holds 750 to 1,150 guests. It has a souvenir boutique, a private celebrity lounge, studios for photo shoots (anything from *Playboy*'s Girls of Cabaret Royale to in-house ads), kitchens serving the "four-star" twenty-four-hour restaurant, dressing rooms, tanning rooms, lockers, showers, administrative offices, executive suites, and an outdoor fountain patio where guests enjoy live bands, free kabobs, and shimmying bare hostesses during the "luau happy hour." Despite its size, it doesn't exude the Magrittean incongruity of the post–oil boom, I. M. Pei–designed Dallas buildings looming against the traveling white country clouds. The Cabaret hacienda has charm. A cobbled shaded courtyard leads through massive wooden doors to a cool lobby of stone. Ochre and sepia walls are decorated by bronze murals. Crystal doors open to the main floor. A Colonial marble staircase winds from the cashier's oak niche (the sign reads "No Guns Please") to a VIP lounge that overlooks the stage. Each dancer performs two main stage shows, two solos on baby grand pianos, and a final one on the VIP stage upstairs. The entry fee is $10 to $25. The dress code is limited to formal wear, or rugged jeans accessorized by a $1,500 ten-gallon hat, snakeskin boots, or gold cuff links.

The darkened floor mills with kittenish women in open raincoats, business suits, pearls, satin gowns, jeweled panties, diamond belly studs. "Class" is part of every big club's success recipe. "We take these girls and in five months we make them into ladies," Nina explains, tottering busily on her stilettos. "We all uphold an image here, like in Disneyland." I dine in the VIP lounge among solemn bland-faced Asian or black men in wrinkle-free suits and loud groups of rumpled white conventioneers.

The Dallas clubs contribute hundreds of millions a year in liquor taxes to the Texas economy—vast public revenues spawned from ten thousand women's naked bodies. This I learn from Jack, C.R.'s new owner, a lawyer in a glossy double-breasted suit and tie, polished loafers, tweezered mustache, and ear stud. He is mild, unruffled, sternly handsome. His grin exudes the cunning of self-made millionaires. His basic profession is mythopoeia. Like a sports coach, Jack's main job is to convince his staff and clients that they are the *best* staff and clients. "I have intelligent girls," he tells me spiritedly, as if brains were the merchandise men chose his club for. "*Playboy*'s college spread features a Cabaret dancer who's an SMU student." Do they recite poetry? I ask. Jack laughs.

The catch-22 for any owner is that customers must buy into a fantasy of him as the guy who gets the money *and* the girls; and at the same time, the outside world—the parents, politicians, bankers, law enforcement and IRS agents—must be assured that, like a Hollywood movie star, he's not the persona he portrays at work but middle-of-the-road Jack. Everyone who works in clubs, from strippers to bouncers, tries to pull off this trick. It's hardest for the owner. He can't join a country club because wives don't want their husbands playing golf with him and politicians cannot be seen with him. Yet inside the parameters of the club, every man wants to be his friend. He must cultivate upstanding citizens with free drinks and chummy attention, and hire local cops for protection, even though they snub him outside. He is a court jester who humbles himself for profit, a self-satisfied "martyr" to capitalist democracy.

Jack has invited two dancers to dinner so I can interview them. "Patsy has been to modeling school," he says. Patsy's lash-barred jaded eyes reflect nothing. A potent narcissism envelops her like a numbing cloud. She is twenty-four and satisfied with herself: "I am thirty-four, twenty, thirty-four," she whispers by way of introduction. Despite the high volume of the jarring music, all the professionals prefer to whisper.

Like most strippers, Patsy and Anka explain that they are doing this temporarily and are "getting out in five or six months." Both girls, presumably the cream of Jack's crop, insist this isn't "who they are." Anka has a small business in Colorado she manages for half the year. She tells me over and over, as if to convince herself: *Money justifies everything. I'm my own boss. This is real life. You can't look after anybody but yourself. We make more than the clients."* She's hard and cynical in a down-to-earth way. Tall, efficient, Swiss-born, Anka is proud to have done away with little feminine softnesses, romantic bonds, and her past. She doesn't speak to her family, whom she sees as potential leeches of her fortune. She's a career woman and has time or need for little else.

Patsy bought a $120,000 house at twenty-two, and may quit at twenty-five (in five months), so she'll "still have her whole life ahead"; but she wants to save $50,000 first, so she may retire at twenty-seven; but she also wants to pay off her mortgage (twelve more years on the job) so she can be secure for life. Patsy tells me she prayed to God to show her a path out of this job, and then told a customer about it, who said: "You like money, you like houses, why don't you get a real estate license?" She now says that was God's reply. She pulls her long silky blond hair away from her waxen face, and her lazy eyes hold mine. "A miracle," she nods. She doesn't have any tangible plans for following up on this divine message.

While we talk, Anka glances over the VIP balcony at the main floor. At one point she matter-of-factly announces, "I see business down there; sorry, I must go do business," and, like a cordial but committed shopkeeper, she picks up her gold-chained pocketbook and struts off with lofty confidence in her shaky heels and clingy cocktail gown. With no visible trepidation she disassociates from the fact that "business" involves her taking off all but a few millimeters of gingham fabric, running her hands over her genitals, unraveling her tits on men's faces, and crawling across strangers' laps. "Business is our mission," Nina confides. "We make sure no one working here forgets it."

On my way out that night, I meet the Cabaret's wiry Arab floor manager at the main exit. His smile is strained; his young creased face looks at home only in derision. "Most of these girls were abused kids," he tells me, his steely eyes steadfastly surveying the room, "so this is familiar to them; they think they want money, power, revenge, but what they want is to be treated like scum. They all need schooling, including a crash course in attitude adjustment. A level temperament and an ability to leave their problems at home is the only thing the stars have over the rest. My job is to keep them all in line, make sure they show up and don't throw too many tantrums. Girls apply for work every night, but we're always on the lookout for happy ones." Suddenly there is a violent commotion at the door; he springs toward it like a threatened boxer, and a tall, wily bouncer gingerly blocks my view.

The next day I secretly visit Tracy, a Cabaret dancer, at her bare downtown apartment. Her bathrobe trails open over her nudity and I gaze at the white walls to discourage her exhibitionism. I presume exposing herself is both habit and self-defense. She flaunts her tan, shakes her wet hair, stretches her aerobicized tendons, slaps her butt. Eventually she gives up her power play and puts on her tights, and I help her carry her dry-cleaned costumes out to her red sports car. Her unwarranted erotic poses continue all afternoon, pestering me like a nagging question. I remain reserved, suspicious of what a girl socialized in the netherspace of men's clubs might take for sociable behavior.

We drive through naked, dusty countryside dotted at wide intervals with forbidding, smoke-glassed industrial skyscrapers; clusters of fenced, garreted condos; shingled one-story houses; and Baptist churches that resemble fast-food outlets. This scattering of odd man-made exclamation points can't mask the flatness of the land. The locals rarely venture outside these climate-controlled structures that look forcefully plunked down on the terrain like model exhibits of interplanetary colonization. In the car, Tracy is raving about the Galleria, a mammoth mall that houses ice-skating rinks and refabricates the "charm" of the USSR in Epcot aesthetic. Her private life centers there and at the Grand, a movie theater consortium of twenty-three screens, stadium-sized amphitheaters, parking-lot golf carts, and arcades of virtual war games.

We eat at Paul's Porterhouse Steaks next to the Cabaret. The waiters, their boots echoing on the ranch-house floor like in old Westerns, serve us buckets of stained meat. All around us, women with bouffant hair, clattering heels, cinched waists, and breasts flaunted like artillery chirp empathetically with tightly clad, belt-buckled men. The men, accommodating and well-mannered, noisily praise the women's looks. Everyone is drenched in cologne.

"I don't like wrestling with clients or lathering them in the shower," Tracy is saying, her perky eyes turning steely. "But I earn more shaking my money maker than most doctors, professors, and mayors. Guys spend hundreds of dollars a night on me, like my dad used to spend on booze on payday. I hate any memory of poverty. All I have to do now is wiggle my tits and I have no fear. I buy something new every day. If I want a fur coat, I call Joe Schmo and tell him. If I feel like the Bahamas, some client can't wait to take me, and I won't even fuck him. So I've no qualms about it. The fact is the 'male gaze' doesn't touch me. I'm feeding on it like a leech."

I ask if she meets with social prejudice. "Sure. I net a hundred thousand dollars a year and some assistant VP at the bank who makes thirty thousand and has two kids and a mortgage treats me as a credit risk. But that's not enough to make me want to be a receptionist. When I hold a regular job, I feel used. I quit dancing, but I missed the ego trip. I went through attention withdrawal. Stripping is a drug. Once you get the bug, you can't shake it off." *Who* is she outside the fantasy? "I've no idea," she says. "I live in the club. I'm just like any other workaholic." So her only friends are coworkers? "I don't need friends. This is dog eat dog. I lock my money or they'll steal it. I don't reveal how much I make. Strippers look for what they can get out of everyone. We have little girl voices and sit on men's laps and never grow up. I talk to *you* because I need you to like me. It's how strippers are." Her voice and her gaze are affectless and indifferent; her body stays in working pose, tits and ass protruding in an *S*.

The Cabaret's main rival is The Men's Club—part of a chain of clubs in Houston, Charlotte, Reno, Guadalajara, and Mexico City. It is located near the Residence Inn where, in March

1996, two teams of suburban police, on the pretext of responding to a noise complaint, banged on the door of the suite where Michael Irvin, star player of the Dallas Cowboys, was snorting cocaine and watching two Men's Club strippers have sex, as he had frequently done before. What caused the ensuing fall from grace not only of Irvin but of the city's legendary team was a tip from a jealous cop who was the boyfriend of one of the strippers involved. The cop ended up in prison, convicted of putting out a contract on Irvin's life. The scandal gave a glimpse into the underside of Dallas's golden clubs.

The cabdriver who takes me to Men's, a fifty-year-old man in a T-shirt that says "Da Boys," warns me, "They got topless women in there," in an urgent tone, as if we still lived in a century when a dressed female would be morally compromised by the proximity of a naked one. At the entrance a prominent sign reads "Proper Attire Required," like those posted outside monasteries. The cashier, her bustier bursting with squished silicone, explains that I'm not "allowed in unaccompanied (by a man)." I argue with her at first, then have the presence of mind to imply I'm shopping for work. A cluster of broad-faced jovial bouncers surround me like bodyguards. They let me in, but not before one of them, incredibly, takes me aside to whisper: "I hope you know there're topless women in there."

The Men's Club is a mansion with cavernous blue-lit rooms, lush carpets, bright stages, upholstered wingback chairs, wait staff in fishnets, and pliable chinalike women churning pneumatic pelvises clockwise. Club beauty is bionic and predictable, the product of tanning lamps, treadmills, surgeons, and computerized lights. Clarity, harmony, rotundness, rosiness, lumpiness, seem extinct. The female body has undergone a phenomenal public transformation here: it has become an exactingly judged performance machine.

"Hi, I'm Lloyd," a stocky neighbor addresses me over the din, chewing on a pork chop. "What brings *you* here?" Human nature, I say awkwardly. A lanky brunette wipes his pudgy fingers daintily, then starts dry-humping him in what strikes me as a comical replay of seventh-grade sex. "Every so often one of them can fake it," Lloyd tells me, flashing a disillusioned smile fraught with crow's-feet at me. "It keeps me young." It seems offensive that he addresses *me* and ignores the thonged brunette who assiduously genuflects to his lap like a trained pet. "Sex is a social construct," he informs me in the manner of an experienced tour guide, spaciously hugging his armchair. "Sex is barter. I always say: I don't make love, I make equity." A minute later he adds, "I pain to see any business opportunity go unexplored. This here is Heather."

Heather is bouncing hard, lashing her hair at his crotch like a broom, to scant attention. I try to imagine what I would feel, if I were a man, at the sight of women bending lower and lower before me as I inspect their disembodied mammal asses; I might sense that what they are selling is not anatomy but their freedom to be anything but a glowing protruding butt; and I might enjoy *that*. "I come here for the illusion of never being at a loss," he explains. Heather grabs the $20, pulls up her halter dress in almost modest haste, smiles coquettishly, murmurs in his ear, and strides off, her neck high, her apathy perfectly mirroring his. "Some girls have a genetic makeup that makes them strippers," Lloyd chats, watching Heather whip off her halter perfunctorily over another slack-jawed man, like a gentleman of another era would watch a cotton picker toil. "It's not moral. It's chemical. They're born strippers. They're incompetent outside a club. Statistics and case histories all show strippers are frigid, sadistic, infertile, antisocial, nymphomaniac, drug-addicted, alcoholic, or mentally ill. They have unstable personalities and inferior home lives. Economic necessity isn't the reason for stripping—it's inborn. Money is the facilitator—the icing."

I arrange to meet Heather at Electrique, her favorite store, which sells studded Brazilian thongs, PVC, T-backs, pasties, hot pants—class-act uniforms, she calls them. In daylight, Heather's razor-sharp cheekbones give her long face a harsh, drawn-out expression; unadorned, her heavy-lidded eyes look insomniac. She commends my hips, using the stock crude standards of male lust, and I suggest I "use" them.

"You have to *spend* money to make money," Heather instructs me, scouting rows of money suits. Strippers have an educating streak. "Killer costumes get the money, cars, condos. A suit must be snug and dressy. Neons, reds, blues, aren't affected by club lights," she advises, heaping a motley pile on the counter. "We get fleeced in this business: fifty-dollar late fines, ten-dollar tips to the staff, ten-dollar fee for makeup and hair in the club—that's the *real* exploitation!" Heather insists she's proud to be commodifying her erogenous zones. I ask if her pride stems from feeling unattainable—like the perverse pride of a guy whose wife is a *Playboy* centerfold. She says it stems from pulling in a grand a night.

Later, as we drive by JFK's fatal grassy knoll, Heather clarifies: "I'm turned on by myself. Stripping is my compulsion. A shrink explained it to my parents; he said it's my recognition of a lack of autonomy. The club is safe. I used to take off my clothes as a kid in front of my dad. I showed my breasts to the boys in junior high. I undressed in front of my window, ripped off my shirt in dance clubs; it was getting dangerous. So I'm grateful for my job: I can live off my monomania."

She's looking bored, as strippers do. I saw her hustle and bust her ass, I say. Doesn't that drain her emotionally? She gives me a mercenary smile. "To meet men and talk and dance is emotional; to charge one dollar a minute is business. When I work, I don't think. I sort of die. It's like yoga: I don't think about the guys, I think 'turn-look-lick lips-bend right-left.' It's automatic. It's nothing." Does she retain her self-respect as she dances? "It's acting," she insists. But she always plays the same part, and that can blur the borders between reality and fantasy, I say. I think strippers are robbed of their chance for a normal social adjustment. "Some nights, after a bachelor party, when guys get the pack mentality and act like their dollar makes them God, I go home and throw up. But, really, I dance for *myself*. Strippers are their own voyeurs. We have male minds. We *get* the male stereotypes. Most of us were tomboys. Most of us are dykes. And that's the goal of feminism, to give women freedom to experience everything like men do. *We* are the real feminists."

The Lodge Bar & Grill is a new backwoods-guy Dallas super club with a heliport, game trophies, roughly cut cedar walls, a giant stone fireplace, and a stage made of massive rocks. A local writer friend and I sit in a faux-frontier alcove away from the stage auction. The Lodge's "minimum 100" girls parade by in gloweringly eye-catching attire, resembling plastic idols, kitschy idealized icons designed to exorcise mortality. Their halfheartedness enhances the ritualism. Their glistening bodies function thoroughly irrespectively of their distracted faces, which appear to be daydreaming. This staggering divide between mind and flesh is as wide and unchallenged as the staunchest puritans would want it.

"I don't understand the appeal of lap dances," my friend says. "They're fake, and they reinforce repression. It's an assembly line." She's never been to a club before. It's a *representation* of sex, I say, like porn; a replay of the primeval struggle between penis and pussy, translated into the struggle between the authority of money and the power of alluring flesh. In the modern strip club, money has replaced masculine traits desirable in millennia past—virility, musculature, agility, courage, honor. A man's wallet is his penis. Wealth is perennially potent; it even resolves male anxieties of size and anatomy. Strip clubs offer every man, from every walk of life, the same fantasy, and booty equal to what he can afford. "So the fun is psychological," my friend says, "and stems from knowing that pussy is subject to money." The long colorful history of men paying women to be courtesans is rooted in the reflex that powerlessness is sexy, I say. This is a bacchanal turned inside out. But the rigorous physical restraint required of men for this unconsummated sexual rapport can give men a sense of power and mastery over nature that's pleasurable. The freedom from disease, stigma, remorse, is also pleasurable.

My friend is indignant because the one job in which women can make more money than men is self-objectification. She insists stripping contributes to larger systemic gender inequalities, and that the strippers' financial power comes at an enormous moral price. She wants to pull the dancers aside and tell them to get less debasing jobs (in boutiques). I want her to buy dances and tell them. But money makes her uncomfortable here. She even makes me buy our drinks by credit card, so we won't touch cash. Meanwhile, the dancers give us encouraging glances, their smiles momentarily unglued and conspiratorial, relieved of the customary "I dare you to not tip me" look. One shows us a poster ("Sex, Sales, Success") and gleefully stutters: "Nice, huh?" I smile back. "Don't patronize them," my friend complains. "Who do you side with, the guys or the gals? Have you even decided who you're writing this *for*?" I don't see how I can take sides, when each side relishes the defeat of the other. All I can do is enumerate the broken fantasies.

On my last night in the Cabaret the Bulls are playing the Knicks in the finals, winning 84 to 81. A buxom blindfolded black girl with cash bulging from her G-string bends her knees and opens her legs toward a pit of noisy men as Michael Jordan dribbles on the big screen behind her. Melissa Etheridge is crooning. I sit at the bar with Melanie and Lisa, two strippers from Connecticut who are working in Dallas while it's too hot for Mexico. They've been friends since kindergarten. "I'm a staunch feminist," Lisa announces in a hyperurban tone. She's short, hardy, and bountiful—large breasts, large pecs, large thighs, waist-long bleached tresses. "No one tells me what to do with my body. I leave men hanging; I treat men like garbage. That's women's lib. It doesn't compromise me more than any other job would. Everybody sells a part of themselves to succeed in this world." It's the revenge of the sex object.

Lisa studied painting in college. Her father writes for *Business Week:* "He's so straight I had to turn pro to own my sexuality, because he raised me sexophobic." In her sophomore year she took up dancing at her boyfriend's urging. "When he dared me to try dancing," she motors away, "I was terrified; I agreed to do it for a night to face my fear. I stayed. It was healing. No-nonsense bump and grind. Then the club was bought out by a chain, they tore down the runway, built four stages, had eight women up at a time; we were mechanical bulls. But I was hooked to the money. I got fired because my butt was too big. I was making shitloads of money, but a boss got on my bad side. The big clubs are run by Nazis. They treat us like cattle. They're bankrolled by the Mafia. My boyfriend worked there unofficially, luring customers to bet on sports events. Girls had to sleep with the bosses' friends for free; they were guys you didn't say no to, if you didn't want to disappear."

Melanie is doelike, frail-boned, soft-spoken, with green unrattled eyes and dewy skin. During the day, she works on her fiction. "I started dancing after a bad breakup," she tells me. "I was down on myself and men, so I filled an application. The club was creepy. One guy always took me and a waitress to the VIP room, paid us $600, and had her feed me Milky Way bars across his lap, spank me, and yell, 'You're so fat!'" She chortles, her long gaunt body peculiarly unguarded, her wide eyes unquestioning. Lisa cuts in: "Most guys don't want Barbies, they want pigs; they're coked or boozed out of their minds and can't even see us; they buy our g-strings to sniff, like dogs. Clubs are roach-infested. Poles aren't cleaned between crotch swipes. There's nothing between you and filth.

"When I started working," she goes on, "I developed vaginal lock. The doctors can't cure it. Men get trapped inside me like dogs in heat. So *this* is my sex life: being a piece of meat. Safe sex. If I do a line of coke, I'll even give hand jobs. It's like sewing." But her body is warning her, I say. This is a far cry from the healing, empowering, feminist experience she described at first. Her body wants out. Why doesn't she go back to painting, to pleasing *herself*? "How little you know, Eurydice," Lisa says cynically. "You think you're outside looking in, but you're in the zoo with the rest of us."

This is what I've learned about the inner workings of strip clubs: strippers embody America's trademark materialist values. Their bodies are commodities used in transactions among the male club owners and customers; as such, strippers are capitalist instruments for male social bonding, their sexuality a matter of pure exchange value. The properties of their bodies are suppressed, transformed into objects of circulation among equally suppressed and objectified men. In a strip club, both the women and the men remain implacably distant from their actual physical instincts, as the libido becomes an essentially economic pleasure: the desire to accumulate goods.

The social service strip clubs perform is not primarily sexual. They cater less to the carnal excesses of the body than to the excesses that occur when the lust for individual power becomes greater than the volatile passions of the flesh. The club is the little man's revenge: it alleviates his stress of being controlled by constricting institutions, politics, technologies, mores; it enables him to feel part of the controlling elite. Within the limits of the club bureaucracy, he can dismiss or cheer bimbos, feel self-reliant, show off his financial prowess, and find refuge from reality in the presence of pumped-up females aping the primal customs of desire. Men work from childhood on so that, cash in fist, they can stare into an unknown woman's vagina without repercussions, without being stricken by God and Mom and Uncle Sam. Strippers may be mechanical orbs, pussy robots, symptoms of a world increasingly dependent on simulations and visual stimuli, that arouse consumers the way advertisements do; but they are also tokens that vindicate men for years of private humiliations, rejections, and failures.

Men drop by the bar and ask how come I'm the only non-working woman here. I *am* working, I say, and show my tape recorder. A disheveled, red-faced computer executive in suit jacket and sneakers introduces himself as Job and quotes the *Iliad* on lust and war. He says he "loves" strippers: "I take them out to lunch, buy them gifts; they're better than shrinks or priests, they pass no judgment. They liberate me from sexual oppression." He has a wife and two kids he "loves," who are his "greatest achievement." "My wife prefers me coming here than to a bar where I might meet a 'real' woman," he adds. "It's my hobby: other men take up sports; I subscribe to *Exotic Dancer Bulletin.*"

By now a dozen curious men blockade me. "Life has become an experiment. Relationships have become negotiations we must work through," Job complains. "*These* girls don't expect men to do everything; in fact, they expect men to do nothing. That's the draw. This isn't about sex; it's *healing.* It gives me balance and confidence. Sure, it's addictive. But my psychic health is worth any money."

This is how I understand it, I tell him gently: Outside, cars honk and he breadwins and socialpillars. Ten bucks later, naked women wrap their legs around him, and there can be no surprises. He pays to be sure women won't slap his face and won't tell him to go fuck himself; they'll call him honey and touch his neck and hair like when he was a boy. He can let go, and still be in control; have his apple pie and eat it, too.

"God bless America," someone tells me. Some of the men listening laugh. Many have trouble staying focused. They pass around cigars. Their eyes dart uneasily. "Nature has bestowed on women a precious gift," someone slurs. "Unfortunately, most women don't know how to use it. All women should exploit their influence; then we wouldn't come here. If women understood their own power, the whole world would be moral."

I say morality requires sexual literacy. This instantly endears me to the crowd. I say desire and fantasy are necessary parts of a healthy life. They clap. I say power is a trap, the bait cast by gods bent on staging moral tragedies. They order a round of drinks. Then they clamor like agitated frat boys, noisily pleading with me to table dance for them.

Cincinnati:
Intercourse by Numbers

"My dear lady, this is a list / Of the beauties my master
has loved / A list which I have compiled. / Observe, read
along with me. / In Italy, six hundred and forty; / In Germany, two hundred and thirty-one; / A hundred in
France, in Turkey ninety-one; / But in Spain, already one
thousand and three!"

Mozart, Don Giovanni

*The bottomless search for psychosexual satisfaction through
quantities of body parts that I saw in strip clubs was a theme I
faced again soon after my return from Dallas, when a friend
called in despair: his wife found a photograph of a busty
bikinied stripper tit-choking him; he wanted me to convince her
of his loyalty and good intentions. So I flew to Cincinnati where
my friend is an architect, and dealt with the drama as best I
could, and there I met my friend's mentor in adultery, a surgeon
named Buck. Buck offered to make a clean breast of his sex life
to me. He wanted to risk showing himself to a woman truthfully
for once, and then examine the results, in order to see what he
had been protecting himself from. He understood that my professional capacity excluded me from the condition of sexual
prey in which he put the rest of womankind, minus his wife. But
honesty is a potent aphrodisiac and he couldn't help trying to
incorporate me into his sex life.*

*D. H. Lawrence said human beings are made up of the "mob-
self," who mindlessly acquiesces in conventional opinions, and
the "individual-self," who is capable of original and subtle*

rebellion. In Ohio, I realized that leading double lives is how conventional people fight a monolithic and monotonous society. I got the impression that loving, clean, well-meaning people who work nine to five and eschew unanswerable questions are implicitly working overtime to destroy their society. This is how societies change. The reason our most common rebellion is sexual in nature is that sexuality has been treated as a dirty secret, by decree of this society, for so long, it has become second nature to hide it, and to make use of the secrecy. From an early age we learn to treat our sexual experience as taboo, to euphemize and falisfy it. As a result, much more often than not, however unreasonably, sex feels like an insubordination, the breaking of some ineffable rule. So sex is the realm where social aberrations most easily flourish. But even our littlest lies deceive our own sense of reality.

Don Juan is our modern archetype of raw sexuality—he is avenging satyr, Dionysian fertility symbol, tomcat, superstud, and a criticism of social hypocrisy. Driven by a rapacious, morally uncontaminated libidinal urge, he is equally drawn to young and old, sharp and dim, lady and maid, virgin and whore, blonde and brunette. The least twinge of desire sends him into the most elaborate and reckless quests for its satisfaction. His is a life of insatiable entropy.

The original poem, "Don Juan, the Libertine of Seville and the Stone Guest," written by Tèrsot de Molina in 1630 (whose text fired the imaginations of Mozart, Molière, Byron, Balzac, Musset, Bernard Shaw, and many others), focuses on the antagonism between the philandering Don and the ghost of a dishonored father whom he's killed in a duel. The ghost haunts him. The Don mocks it, continues his cuckolding escapades, even makes a statue of the ghost to decorate his garden, and derisively invites it to dinner. At the climax the statue comes to life, warns him that his time is up, and asks him to repent.

The Don refuses and joins the damned in eternal hell. The statue represents the fixed (petrified) morals of the society, which prevail by a might the Don should have recognized—the validity of numbers—as the covenant of the multitudes. But deep down Don Juan knows the numbers can fail us; the ideal of an enlightened majority has been historically elusive—which is why, in addition to guaranteeing the rights of the majority, democracy must guarantee the rights of any peacefully dissenting minority (which is the only way to achieve an enlightened majority). In this sense, Don Juan is an inveterate Emerson-Dewey democrat.

For the women he seduces, Don Juan represents both a return to animality and a challenge to domesticate an untamed manhood; he provides them with unequivocal worship, danger, delight, despair—with possibilities that conventional civilization excludes. In the eyes of men, he is both a menacing sex-thief and the inner predator all men would love to let free. For the society at large, he represents an immature violator of public mores, community standards of decency, a degenerate libertine unfettered by common inhibitions, a ravenous automaton that must be stopped. In the 1990s, he is a classic sex addict, a helpless victim.

Cincinnati is an overcast, big-boned town, with derelict thirties buildings, chimneys spewing white smoke over the Ohio River, gaudy Art Deco skyscrapers, a block-long Masonic temple, a baseball team known for its racist owner, and an art museum famous for demonizing Mapplethorpe. "How many Cincinnatians does it take to screw in a lightbulb?" the day's copy of *The Cincinnatian* reads. "Only one, but we'd prefer you didn't use the word 'screw.'" In rush hour, the downtown is a site of work ethic gone totalitarian. The few panhandlers are scrubbed and courteous. The shadiest alleys look empty and inviting. The city elements stand eerily in place, one-dimensional props waiting to be populated by human passions. Ironically, I'm here to meet a sex addict.

Buck Mulligan (a pseudonym he chose) is a happily married forty-year-old surgeon who has been secretly bedding an average of ten women a month for the past ten years. He is currently seeing four nurses and a fellow doctor at work, and picking up random strippers and strangers after work. (Last week he followed an unknown woman to a crack house, where he was attacked by hoods.) It's male vanity ("egotestical," he calls it) that makes Buck share his Casanovian secret life with me. His male friends think his exploits are the epitome of masculinity. Buck himself doesn't believe he is an addict. Experts say that most addicts don't, until they hit rock bottom.

"I wanna be dashing and suave for you," Buck worries when we meet, "but my life is normal and boring. I fuck every woman I can, so what?" I say I'm here to find out what enables him to rise before dawn, sip his coffee, glance at the paper, drive ten miles to work, cut people up for ten hours a day, save a life, then get a massage, fuck the masseuse, go home, cook, fuck his wife, go to a bar, fuck a stranger, and wake up the next day for another round of breaks-and-entries.

"Surgery is the ultimate penetration," Buck explains as we traverse the big brown hospital in the eye-stabbing light of early morning, accompanied by the drone of vacuum cleaners. "I compare it to scuba diving. I go in, and there's nothing left to hide. I'm involved with the core of someone's body. Like sex, it's about gaining trust." He points out a nurse in sensible flats and a peroxide perm: a recent conquest.

The threshold of the operating area leads to a stunning sterility. The air is cold, the faces sedate, the voices monotonous. Surgery, the most intimate human interaction, takes place in the most anonymous of settings. I put on pistachio-colored scrubs, shoe slips, shower cap, a mask. So you battle death both on hospital beds and hotel beds, I say. "I battle degrees of suffering," Buck says. "My only chance against death is getting a healthy twenty-two-year-old who's just been shot. The rest is buying time, playing games." Through his anti-HIV face shield, he dabs wintergreen on his nose so as not to smell the fetid bowels. On the white bed, a woman lies under an anesthetic mask, her belly and abdomen layered with stick-on plastic. A sheet separates her head from her body, making it look harmlessly decapitated. The key to Buck's world is acute objectification; the prone woman is a conceptual problem.

The surgeons slash and burn and chat about CNN. The stench of burning flesh seeps into everything, as they cauterize millimeter after millimeter of yawning, filleted skin to control the bleeding. "There is a rhythm between me and the organs," Buck whispers, performing quick, minute incisions into a bed of bloated meaty innards while I stand inches away from a live pulsing human liver. "A liver is so beautiful. I'd operate with bare hands if I was allowed. I like surgery because I touch people; it's hands-on, like in woodshop. Same with sex." He appears oblivious of the psyche at hand; and yet, if she were awake, he would treat her with charm and intensity.

Afterward, Buck calls his wife to pretend that he'll be on ER all night, so we can hit the town. He feels alive at the prospect. "Without this pursuit of sex," he says, "I'd be celebrating my suburban death right now. Sex is a validation. Maybe I do it so people will say, 'You're a *good* guy, you fuck well.' I know my work goals twelve years ahead. I know the ten days I have off in the next two years. With sex, I'm allowed to be unpredictable. My daily life *needs* an element of chaos."

We first drop by a bookstore-café droning with the chatter of coy slackers. Buck's gaze catches onto a starry-eyed, bumbling high schooler, and he lunges to talk to her. Hunger lights up his face. Watching him operate, I can deconstruct his attraction: a big boyish face; a concerned, smooth-like-a-bullet voice; a titanic body—a white-picket-fenced house in himself, a roof to hide under in the rain; and everything that he is culminates in one central aspect: he wants to be wanted.

The high schooler has a date for tonight, so they exchange

phone numbers and we move on. Across the street, a big black woman in a vinyl jacket and straightened hair rushes to a lone graffiti-framed 7-Eleven with an urgent stride. Like a hound, Buck gets a spring in his step and offers to showcase his sex-baiting technique on her. We haven't even seen her face. I realize how indiscriminate, even cold-blooded, his appetite is, a testosterone-driven maelstrom. He calls it human curiosity.

"I've been with Turks, Chinese, Latinas; I learn from all. I experiment. I pendulum in, figure out all I want, pendulum out. If I say 'I'm gonna get fucked now,' I can just grab a woman and dance with her, and she'll take me home and put me through the wringer. It's that easy. Because I'm good at cutting through the rubbish and saying, 'I want you.'" He can be blind to everything but the lay, and that's what makes an effective Lothario. And he can see beauty in unlikely places. "One feature for me is enough: a nose, an eye, even if the rest is ugly. I've slept with a woman for her neck alone." He makes me wonder if objectification isn't the ultimate manifestation of democracy.

At a nearby bar, facing a deafening mediocre band, Buck sips his Bloody Mary hawk-eyed. "You don't look like you belong here," he suddenly tells a slim thick-haired girl with a large tantalizing mouth and tight jeans. "You belong somewhere far from here." But his eye has already located a better target, a snotty dressed-up blonde sitting with a herd of preppy corporate clones. "I'm gonna go tell that blonde what she's doing is empty," he tells me. "I need to surprise her, shake her up. I don't know if she'll leave with me right away, but that's the risk I take. Sometimes it takes time; women start out thinking I'm scheming. So I need time to talk. That's the bottom line." "You need to leave these people you're with," he unceremoniously tells the blonde. She faces him in mildly offended disbelief, then smiles, interested, and listens on; soon, her mind is under a form of anesthesia.

Language is the magic pill that separates sex from plumbing, and Buck uses it as the lure to his vanishing act. "I could disappear in you," he tells her, sly enough to make himself vulnerable. His medical training has familiarized him with the importance of bedside codes that earn confidence. His success both as a doctor and as a philanderer stems from his psychological acuity: he "cares" about his lays in the manner he cares about his sick; he doesn't boast, he focuses on them. Deftly, sagaciously, devotedly, he signals that he sees in them what no other man has: inspiration, wit, beauty, passion. So what if he does it to every female he meets? He enables women to feel admired, treasured, and, however briefly, loved. He makes their reality feel fantastic and their dreams real.

Buck trades in hyperbole and politesse. "You *are* desire," he tells me. "She is a genius," he says of a stripper. "*You* are a genius," he says later, revealing the secret of his success: he is not afraid of inviting ridicule. His talk is unabashed because conversation is his mating game. Without words, he would be emasculated. He must convince each woman his lust isn't about him, nor about her entire sex, but only about *her* irresistible charms. Perhaps in the solitude of a night in his conjugal bed he has known moments of terror, but the Buck I meet has no internal mirror or censor, and that is the hallmark of a bona fide seducer. That is the tragicomic essence of Don Juan.

Don Juan's lust becomes his trap *because* he is only in love with himself. So his quest perpetually eludes him: even if he could possess all women simultaneously, he still would not find peace. He forgets this conundrum in the thrill of danger, speed, deceit. He moves about masked, scales balconies, descends ladders, runs on rooftops, finding pleasure in the velocity of change and impersonation. He wears disguises not so much to escape the vengeance of fathers, husbands, judges, as to escape the tedium of sexual repetition. He can't see that what keeps his satisfaction impossible and incomplete is what killed ravishing, lonely, silly Narcissus.

Buck's next stop is a club steeped in red light, owned by a lady in bifocals who leaves her desk to examine me closely.

Jaundiced women in Day-Glo G-strings and sequined paste-ons hover within touch. Surprisingly, I find these dejected refugees of life-next-door in their cheap skimpies authentically sexy, unlike the high-class strippers I have seen. They hang from ballet bars looking catatonic and anemic, saddled with rippling cellulite or pockmarked skin, passing around semi-demented smiles. The audience keeps its gaze fixed on the genitals. "I don't think about anything when I'm here," Buck says. "Of course, all the women are on Valium." I observe him chat up a misshapen gartered waitress. Clearly, like a latter-day Pygmalion, he creates his object of desire as he talks. His verbal prowess, more than the woman-of-the-instant, turns him on. "I like down-and-dirty bars because I can talk the girls into meeting me for a quickie in the alley. I want them to go beyond what they're supposed to do. That's fundamental," he explains.

Buck is also a master of silence. Without the silence he elicits from every woman he sleeps with—from traffic cops to surgeons—he couldn't manage his double life undetected. I find it amazing that all his women agree to play second fiddle to a wife who gains nothing from their silence but a pretense of marital bliss. "We have an unspoken agreement that we're making a limited engagement," Buck explains. "It's pride. No woman wants to be seen as a homewrecking temptress."

I ask about his wife. He loves her—spurred by familiarity and habit, and also guilt and expiation. He needs her as a nun needs her well-worn rosary. His wife is the safety net that lets Buck plunge into the heroic adventures of the outside world without getting lost. But he says that *because* he loves her, their sex can't peak; it inevitably "tapers off into affection." He is cuddly and sweet with her, but his self-esteem is tied to the number of women who want him. Without the testimonies of their love, he feels hollow, unrealized. "Extramarital sex is fragile, insecure, intense. Marriage is too subtle."

Buck's wife is a plucky English-rose-type medical designer.

"We are 'perfectly compatible,' " Buck says. But he laughs patronizingly when I ask if *she*, too, is sneaking out into her own labyrinths to screw unsubtly. Buck adheres to the old dichotomy of wife/madonna and mistress/whore. He feels no compunction about adultery so long as he doesn't hurt his wife—by confessing to her or by abandoning her. "I grew up in a well-off Christian family. I slept with my high school teacher. My first fantasy was being the only male on a women's planet. I felt like a dickhead who would go to hell for this. In my teens, I suffered worlds for fucking. After I had therapy, I stopped reacting to the world with guilt. I don't hate myself. I can't afford to."

Has he ever resolved not to cheat again? "Once, my wife's best friend came by to drop off a book and gave me a blow job, just like that. That was scary. But I can't say no: the experience is too essential. Besides, the consequences of all those affairs, in terms of retributions, have been *nothing*"; he sounds almost regretful. The possibility of being caught heightens the excitement and instability he longs for. Fear is part of his elixir: he seeks what he fears for the thrill of the fear more than the thrill of possessing or understanding it. Examine your lust, I suggest; basically, a disease is an uncontrolled hunger. "I guess I have a sex wish. And what you are doing to me now is surgery—cutting through me, getting it all," Buck meekly answers. "The difference is, I can feel it." He starts crying.

We're back at my hotel, having a late dinner. All around us useful-looking men bustle about in matching laundered suits and manners. They order drinks and supper and sit through boastful sales chats, laughing forcedly, their eyes drifting off to the periphery as if whiling away the time until they are free to unwind their anxiety of being civilized in after-hours diversions. They look like Bucks in the making, or unmaking. Work as salvation from nature is the motto of this tribe.

Next, Buck baby-talks a mistress on the hotel phone and sighs to his wife about the madness at ER. His face becomes a mask of concentrated compassion. The guilelessness of his everyday deceit stuns me. It shouldn't: lying is the very source of his charm; he only tells a woman what she wants to hear. A womanizer can't afford to be honest with himself or the women he pursues. And like any good manipulator, he must momentarily believe his elaborate lies. "Working all this out takes planning, presence of mind," he says, proud as a farmer looking upon a freshly plowed field. "You learn to compartmentalize. You start to coordinate like a general." Is the time and concentration invested in it worth it? "Worth it? People sit home watching TV all the time!" he protests.

We conclude our long night at the seediest venue yet, a Piano Lounge that has no piano, no bouncer, and no cover, just a floor show of unceremoniously raised legs. Men come here to flirt with a nearly naked female while she sips a $10 drink. We meet two diligent identical twins whom Buck has fucked in drunken tandem and who don't remember it. Buck points animatedly toward a mammoth-breasted stripper, vying for her attention. "Sam," he says, winking and waving, "has a crush on me. She just had her breasts done. Twenty pounds per tit. Back muscles of titanium."

When he has sex with these women, does he ever wonder: Who *is* this person? "Going in there, I assume they've been waiting all their lives for me," he cuts me off. And afterward? "I don't hang out and talk to them. In and of itself, sex is shallow. I crave quantity just to convince myself it's real. What I'm seeking is no different from what everyone seeks in life, which is the *meaning* of it. But I don't spend my life contemplating it; I act out," he brags, unknowingly using addict terminology. "Biologically, our bodies are geared to reproduce at the highest possible rate; if we didn't have a conscience, we'd all fuck all the time. A hard-on is the only thing that defies gravity, our only chance to fly." But hasty mechanical reiteration limits the full potential of sex, I say. Love is a great aphrodisiac. It makes even miserable lovers seem sublime. All *he* gets is the Burger King of lust. "Love takes up time; and I don't want to trifle with women's hearts; I don't want any *responsibility*." I think Buck's desire is never used up because its object is mute, pornographic. What relieves its monotony is quantitative acceleration. The tragedy of libertinage is that it claims nature for its justification, yet its pleasure is mechanized: most debauchery is actually an *overregulation* of the complexities of sexual desire. It's raison d'être is sex-hatred.

It's closing time at the Piano Lounge and Buck is disappointed: he has vowed to "hit" tonight before my prying eyes, but partly because of my intrusive presence he hasn't scored. He won't admit defeat. Back in my hotel, he determinedly calls up and sweet-talks his "reserves." One of them has just got home from a party, and she agrees to meet him in my room. While we wait for her, he sends his wife flowers.

"I just love his spontaneity," the crimson-cheeked peroxided nurse tells me by way of greeting as she drunkenly sits herself on my bed, in an attempt to explain why she is here. Buck shuts her mouth with a probing tongue and pushes her against the headboard, pawing and groping, mumbling that he's missed her and wants to please her. She has no time to ask who I am and I have no advance warning of the lightning-quick penetration that follows. I don't want to draw attention to my presence by moving; I stand in place, still, aloof. One moment I catch her smiling at me apologetically from behind his back, as if saying "Doctor knows best." The next moment she disappears under his sweaty half-clothed mass. He never looks her in the eye. Her face is being mashed against his chest. It all happens fast. He spasms. I don't know if she comes.

Voyeurism in the line of duty doesn't prove as traumatic as I would expect; it's like having a blood test: one prick, and then I can exhale. After all his verbal excess, the sexual act itself is performed in detonating silence. Their mute physical merging carries with it a loss, an undeniable little death; it strikes me that sex of this sort is like the moment when the lights fail onstage; the moment nothingness gapes open.

• • •

At thirty-eight, Jackie has slept with over a thousand men.
With the exception of short periods when, as a student, she
worked for an escort agency to pay for a summer vacation in
Europe and turned five tricks a day, the rest of those hundreds
she's fucked for pleasure. On her last AIDS test, she checked
the one-hundred-or-more-partners-in-the-past-six-months category. When does she find time for so much sex? "Good sex is
hard to find," she replies in a wise-woman tone, updating
Flannery O'Connor. "Especially consistently. I've never felt a
dick inside me I didn't like, but very few make me go back for
a repeat. I'm like an art collector. I make time. I'm an addict."

Jackie is a pert, wholesome blonde in cutoffs, a Mets
T-shirt, and mismatched socks, a hard-core version of Teri
Garr. "I resist the cocktail-circuit look," she says, pointing to
her outfit ruefully. "My mother is a society lady." Growing up,
Jackie cut class and checked herself into a mental asylum to
get out of high school. She ended up working as a bartender,
stripper, drug dealer. At twenty-eight, she joined a band and
married a gay musician. "I don't see him much. I join him on
tour and get to fuck his band members. It's fun; I never know
who it will be that night," she says wistfully and laughs at herself. Besides the band, she has two other "steady" lovers: a
twenty-four-year-old actor she has slept with since he was sixteen, whose mother is her best friend, and a twenty-five-year-
old sometime model who has a wife and kids. "But even boys
get that look of fear of intimacy after sex," she complains.
"Women today know that sex is fun and free, but men still
believe it carries a price—babies, dinners, entanglements,
attachment, the *Last Tango in Paris* syndrome."

Jackie explains that she has sustained dozens of friendships or affairs through the years, but she's never sustained
romantic love. "I have friends I talk to and I have guys I fuck;
it's unnatural to expect anyone to be both." She would still like
an intimate relationship, but she knows the obstacles: the

aforementioned postcoital fear of entrapment men feel that compels her—out of pride and practicality—to reject them emotionally before they do her; her own experience of the failure of monogamy; and her conviction that ownership and power conflicts accompany intimacy, and corrode it.

"I used to feel jealousy eating at my heart when I was in love," she says. "If I thought my guy went with someone on the side, I'd go with four men to get even. I'd have compulsive sex not for me, but to punish him. I went into therapy to learn my *real* reasons for having sex. A lot of it was out of fear, insecurity. I wanted power. I never got it. Now I can get up right after sex, get dressed, and say 'See ya,' without feeling lonely. If I want more from men, I'll crash. So I'm existential about love. I stay single."

Jackie has been in Narcotics and Sex Addicts Anonymous for seven years. "Sex is like drugs: the first time is great, so you look for more. Basically, all addicts want is to feel better. Sometimes I fuck somebody because the silence between us is making me uncomfortable and I have no idea what else to do. Sometimes I just need sex to lighten up. Other times sex feels like I'm shooting coke every night—it leaves me empty, lost, powerless. When all I do is get laid, it's a bad high. But unlike drugs, good sex still works—I feel happy, strong, one with God. I'm such a slave to sex, I'll put it before anything else. I figure it's just sex, it's not like I get a knife and kill people. All I really want is to feel alive." Is sex the only experience of being alive she knows? "It's the only thing in life that engages all of me. Too bad I can't live on it alone." She has devised a system for getting through her daily life: "I sleep with a different person every day for a week as my reward if I've achieved a goal in my life. I have a celebration, guys are scaling my walls. Then I stop, set another goal, and try to keep to myself. I do hate that castor-oil part, but it motivates me."

I ask why most sex addicts are men. "Guys could fuck a headless woman," she says. "Men don't mind faked sex. I think misogyny is at the root of sex addiction. That's why I'm a 'nympho' whereas men are 'playboys.' But unlike most men, I'm picky. I'm attracted to energy, not physical bodies. Most men don't know how to fuck; they think they're blowing your mind, but they've no idea how good it can be; they're into the *idea* of fucking." I'm reminded of Buck's climactic performance. "I'm drawn to men who'd never go to a strip club," she goes on, "mostly skateboarding punk rockers I pick up at concerts or movies—skinny well-hung Tom Waits types. Those guys fuck like machine guns, like shooting speed. We're sex athletes. We push the limit."

How does one distinguish authentic desire from addict desire? "Sex addiction is bad sex. When you fuck and wish you were doing the dishes, when you have forgettable sex again and again, it's 'acting out.' Good sex is when you go so far into annihilation that there's no world, no God, no mind, when you die on some level," she describes, demarcating "good" and "bad" by the yardstick we all use: how much we like it. This experience of annihilation or transcendence is a big part of what society fears about sex. And Jackie's "annihilation" doesn't contradict her own previous interpretation of sex as the feeling of being alive. What she says is that sex can't be defined; at its best, it's a death of logic.

Unfortunately, I point out, this distinction between good and bad sex can only be made after the fact. Is there no way to guarantee good sex except by trying out lovers like data? Can't emotional attachment ensure great sex? "To me, that's an old wives' tale. Good sex is impersonal, like heroin; it makes me feel free, warm, safe, happy, released from the bondage of myself."

Giovanni Giacomo Casanova, author of one of the greatest memoirs in history, was a typical overachiever: while being a compulsive womanizer, he was also a playwright, travel writer, secretary, soldier, preacher, actor, musician, alchemist, founder of a lottery, silk manufacturer, gambler, Freemason, convicted sorcerer, double spy and paid informer, tutor to the Pomeranian Cadet Corps, librarian, translator of the *Iliad,* and collaborator on the *Don Giovanni* libretto. But what is most interesting in Casanova's twelve-volume memoir is his grasp of time and repetition. He lives for variety, for novelty of a limited serial sort: to do the same things with different women. He is driven by the fact that there are more women to be had than he can even imagine. So he lives like a predatory cuckoo clock. Ritualistic repetition is at the heart of addiction: so long as one repeats the same moves, and satisfaction lasts for the length of each repetition, one's physical experience grows increasingly spiritual. While it lasts, a liaison has all of Casanova's ecstatic devotion, even if the Inquisition is after him. But the impetus of his infinitely replicated once-in-a-lifetime romances is not phallic, but poetic: it's the desire to escape time and mortality. Ironically, sex is his bid for eternal life—the other side of a religious quest.

Sex and Love Addicts Anonymous (SLAA) first emerged in the seventies in Boston as an offspring of the Jungian-evangelical AA twelve steps, modified to treat "selfish" compulsive sexual needs. SLAA's *Big Book* bible, based on Dr. Patrick Carnes's pioneer work, came out in 1985. Sex Addicts Anonymous (SAA) was formed at that time by members who found the SLAA model too loose. Today there are over twelve hundred SAA groups meeting in churches and hospitals worldwide.

SLAA defines "sex and love addiction as a progressive illness which cannot be cured but which, like many illnesses, can be arrested. It may take several forms, including a compulsive need for sex, extreme dependency on one person, and/or a chronic preoccupation with romance, intrigue, or fantasy."

The 1994 edition of *Diagnostic and Statistical Manual of Mental Disorders (DSM-IV)* lists sexual addiction under Sexual Disorder Not Otherwise Specified, and defines it as "distress about a pattern of repeated sexual relationships involving a succession of lovers who are experienced by the individual only as things to be used." The term *sexual addiction* was put on the map in 1983 when Patrick Carnes, a former prison psychologist, published his book *The Sexual Addiction.* He defined sex addicts as people whose sexual behavior had become unstoppable, despite severe consequences such as job loss, family breakdown, and STDs; he offered a twenty-five-question sexual addiction screening test; response in the affirmative to thirteen or more suggests addiction. Many of those questions are disturbingly general: "Have you subscribed to or regularly purchased sexually explicit magazines? Have you ever worried about people finding out about your sexual activities? Has sex been a way to escape your problems? Do you need to have sex or fall in love in order to feel like a 'real man' or 'woman'?"

The Cincinnati SAA meetings are CD (closed discussion), which means I must be a sex addict to attend, so I pose as one. Buck refuses to wear the addict moniker, and is not permitted to accompany me as a friend, since the twelve-step ritual involves denouncing outside support as codependency and standing up alone before strangers to reveal oneself in the humbling ceremonial group terminology: "Hi, I'm Paul and I molested prepubescents." The basic healing method is to treat powerlessness with conscious powerlessness. I introduce myself to the assembly as "helplessly sexual," but I find it hard to act terrified of sex or repentant, and their cheery cult-like fanaticism alienates me.

Paul is my perky SAA sponsor. (A sponsor is an assigned "seasoned and sober SAA" who provides a healthy model for a new member.) He's an athletic, circumspect, impeccably mannered, all-American male who looks like he dislikes his own body fluids. He explains that, unlike SLAA, which lets its members set bottom-line sexual quotas for themselves, SAA prohibits sex or masturbation outside a long-term monogamous relationship: "The goal is to avoid chaos, drama, the loss of boundaries that people bottom out on. Our rule of thumb is SAFE (no Secret, Abusive, Feeling-altering, Empty sex). Ninety meetings in ninety days is our recommended method for starting recovery. Our suffering unites us."

At thirty-one, Paul is the scion of a rich banking family, has a three-year-old son, was molested by an uncle as a child (childhood abuse is considered a classical addiction trigger), and lives in a halfway house sponsored by SAA. Paul is a Level Two addict, an offender. His wife, a social worker who fears that he might molest his own son, has denied him visitation rights. With me, Paul is paternally compassionate and glibly sophisticated, though he scrupulously avoids my gaze.

I ask him to define the difference between addict and nonaddict sex. As I see it, both addict and nonaddict sex stem from the same need to lose ourselves in redemptive pleasure, to forget who we are in quotidian form and remember who we are in our biological core. Paul impatiently objects to my choice of vocabulary. "Nonaddict sex is the result of *spiritual* love and strict monogamy," he lectures. "All the rest is the addiction. Try not to think in extremes. There're pleasures in life that don't involve pathos; self-acceptance is the main one."

Paul belongs to a group of people who attend meetings every day, driving as far as it may be necessary to join their SAA comrades, monitor their progress, and expunge their unacted-upon desires. I ask him if SAA has replaced the confessional. Have the meetings become the addiction?

"You're right," he concedes, "in that we're never free of addiction; if that's your behavior pattern, you must learn to use it for good rather than bad. SAA gives us discipline and makes us accountable. In SAA we watch out for HALT signals—feeling Hungry, Angry, Lonely, Tired; those are the times addicts 'medicate,' take a hit. You get depressed, things go wrong, you act out to get numb, to forget and feel good; then you feel shame and guilt, and you deal with it by wanting to act out again so you won't crash. Or things go well, but you get too tired or too confident, and you thoughtlessly act out, feel horrible, and you go act out again, to punish yourself."

I conclude that we live in an era of moral schizophrenia. Paul's cycle of self-loathing is based on the assumption that casual sex involves a loss of self-control akin to a loss of selfhood. But feeling out of control is not *being* out of control: our genes *want* us to experience desire as a trancelike sexual "powerlessness." Resisting it is hubris. Yet in our day, having divorced sex from procreation, we feel shame for feeling at the mercy of instinct. Ironically, we still see civically meaningless sex as a grave trespass of our social functions.

It's not odd that in a culture promoting both craven self-indulgence *and* draconian self-control, that glorifies translucent nubile exhibitionism *and* genderless professionalism, the need for spontaneous corporeal relief can become a disease. Even as we're urged to consume fathomless pleasures, we're urged to renounce pleasures. In this general breakdown of our ethics, our pleasure can become our punishment: it becomes sex as punishment for sex. Even Patrick Carnes's prototype of a sex addict is someone with a low self-esteem and a "sex negative personal belief system" that stems from associating sex with shamefulness.

Paul concludes: "The first key to recovery is scrupulous honesty. Rationalization is our best and most dangerous tool. Addicts are type-A perfectionists driven to excel. Addicts are among the smartest people on the planet because we learn how to lie and play people from an early age. But we are powerless as individuals and our addiction isolates us. We spend our lives turning and turning, like the earth." Sartre explained addiction as the *absolute* exercise of our freedom of choice, a symptom of our determination to live in the now so completely that we ignore the passage of time marked by our previous resolutions and refuse to be conscious of anything belonging to the past. This temptation to live entirely in the uncontaminated present clashes against our need for a marmoreal stability and a fixed moral center. I tell Paul most people I know fall into this category.

Carnes estimates that 3 to 6 percent of adult Americans are sex addicts. Available research shows that they range in age from nineteen to seventy; most are between thirty-five and forty-five; 81 percent are men, 19 percent women; 90 percent are white, 41 percent married, 23 percent divorced, 63 percent heterosexual, and 38 percent have had postgraduate education. Most addicts are ambitious, willful, disciplined. Their preoccupation with sex is a way to dissociate from stress: casual sex works as an analgesic. Only 16 percent of sex addicts are in recovery—compared to 52 percent for anorexia, 48 percent for alcoholism, 43 percent for nicotine. SAA's therapist manuals list ten types of sex addicts with 114 different behaviors. "Sexual self-abuse" is the second most common compulsion.

Chip is twenty-six, model-beautiful, the lone gay member of Paul's inner group. "Furtive sex is part of gay culture," he coolly asserts. "The more you have, the more respect you get. It's a macho thing." Every few weeks Chip goes to bus station bathrooms and follows any willing man into a stall. A dozen blow jobs later, he takes the train back to his SAA retreat in the throes of remorse. He's a Level One addict—socially harmless. "Sex addiction is like a split personality," he says. "The allure is in the secrecy; the disease involves going undercover. No one close to me would guess I solicit in public toilets. That gives me a power rush, like I'm fooling the world; I get away with it. For years I used sex as therapy: I went to the park whenever I was having a bad day—it was like downing a quick martini. I was so scared of HIV, I'd swear I'd never do it again. The self-hate is the addiction sign. I hated being unable to control it, so I kept going back resolved not to do it, to prove my strength. And I kept failing. As soon as I lapse, I run back to my normal life, but I'm dying inside." He has attended the best thirty-day sex rehab programs in the country, has had round-the-clock counseling, named his every memory, contacted his perpetrators, set his boundaries, taken full moral inventory of himself, accumulated five six-month-sober bronze medallions. He's done his SAA work. "But it's never out of your system," he assures me. "Addiction is like HIV." Chip contracted AIDS during a "relapse" on a vacation in Brazil after a long period of sexual sobriety (successful abstinence from all sexual activity may be followed by "bundling" and then a gradual return to "normal" sex; it is at this transitional point that the treatment usually fails). "No matter what I do, when I'm not in group, I act out. I go about reciting my SAA slogans: 'Let go and let God,' 'This too shall pass.' But sex is my life's lesson, which I will only learn by my death," he adds in an eerily disengaged tone. His tragedy strikes me as an oxymoron.

"Harold C. Lyon, director of federal education programs for gifted children," I read in the day's *Washington Post,* "was sentenced to nine months in jail despite his pleas that he committed three sex-related misdemeanors because he suffers from a mental illness that caused him to be 'addicted to sexual gratification.' " What I detect between these lines is a monstrous coupling: sexual gratification as mental illness. There is no such thing as a rogue anymore: the old roués and yesterday's sociopaths are now biochemically disabled addicts. The concept of sex as mental disorder absolves us of personal responsibility for embarrassing or defiant behavior. It's the castration of Don Juan. "James Cermak's attorney," reads the *Minneapolis Tribune,* "argued that sentencing Cermak for each sex offense would be like sentencing an alcoholic for each drink he takes." According to Carnes, when we have sex, our brains produce dopamine, the same neurochemical that our bodies metabolize from alcohol. This is how sexual obsession qualifies as an addiction, though it involves no chemical use. There are about three hundred chemicals regulating the brain's neurochemistry. We "understand" sixty of them. These naturally occurring opioids (enkephalins and endorphins), first "discovered" by scientists in 1978, are the culprits of the chemical imbalance addicts presumably suffer from. Addicts and experts expect we will soon have the technology needed to cure addiction with a "smart pill"—a Prozac-like serotonin inhibitor—taken for life; to me, it's a moot hope, because (a) *all* sex creates a chemical "imbalance" and (b) so does the lack of it, as millions will testify.

At a time when we are finally in mastery of our natural resources, the needs of our bodies have emerged as the last frontier to tame. So we explain our "helplessness" as a genetic pathology and go about treating it. "Controlling sex addiction with will power is like trying to think away a broken leg," advises SAA's "Twelve Step Recovery" brochure. I'd say the same about sexual need. Peace can only be found in a culturally sanctioned congruency between our primitive and our cognitive urges. If sexual dissatisfaction stems from larger social voids, it may be untreatable within the existing system. We are genetically programmed to be sexually active. We turn "addictive" when our natural impulse is socially hindered or unsuccessfully sublimated. If pleasure remains elusive, the search for it becomes a tyrannical compulsion. SAA's cure-by-abstinence seems self-defeating. As William Blake wrote, "He who desires but acts not, breeds pestilence."

At my next SAA meeting, when I'm asked to "rise and tell my story," I admit I don't "monitor" my intake of pleasure because I think repressed natural desires inevitably mutate and become perverted. I read from SLAA's "Forty Questions for Self-Diagnosis"; question #9: "Have you ever felt that you *had* to have sex?" Everyone has. Question #24: "Do you feel that life would have no meaning without a love relationship or without sex?" From our cradle lullabies onward, we are assiduously trained to espouse this philosophy of romantic success as the key to living happily ever after. Question #3: "Do you feel you need to hide your sexual activities from others?" Most of us are most of the time socially compelled to. My coaddicts say that my "treating sexual need lightly is exactly the root of the problem." They also deplore that I seem intemperately drawn to drama and verbal-emotional highs. "Any unpredictability," they remind me, "leads to acting up." I argue that, without highs and surprises, we will end up fucking like robots. They argue that I desperately need to keep coming back every day for three months.

Americans Abroad: Virgins at Heart

"The mind's road to God always begins in the sexual appetite."

St. Bonaventure

It was the time of year for my annual trip to Europe. By now I was feeling the captive of a collective fever that had kept me moving at a perverse hallucinatory pace, overloading my circuits. Europe gave me instant relief with its sonorous non-English sounds and people whose sex lives didn't matter to me and whose secrets I didn't want to know. I was visiting a dear friend in Rome and on my second day went with her to an expatriates' lunch. The guest of honor was an American monsignor. "Doesn't a monsignor feel the need to have sex?" I asked him, oblivious of the unwarranted psychological invasion I was committing, of how I had mechanically embraced the habit of addressing intrusive questions to strangers and withstanding the vertigo that originates when a person opens up as if it were an unavoidable gust of wind in my path. "If you got the place, I got the time," he joked. This answer was so normal and so shocking to my conventional expectations that I asked to interview him. He accepted. Then I began thinking of sacred edicts and canons and how successfully they had bridled spontaneous sexuality, of the moral myths and symbols that guard society from nature and saddle us intangibly with calumnious inhibitions. I realized I had come to the source of it all; I could end my journey right here, at the latest origin of the morality knot; the place where the ticking clock of the last two millennia had been willfully set by a celibate monk.

Mystics of all traditions have invoked God as a lover who leads them into states of rapture. As an energy that transports us back and forth between the manifest and unmanifest worlds, and promotes the dissolving of the I, sex has always been of interest to priests, shamans, healers. In the pre-Christian world, erotic rites like Sufi zikrs, pagan spring festivals, Hindu Holi, tantric yogic enactments, and ancient Bacchic-Orphic mysteries addressed a basic longing that therapy, recovery, prevention and sex-education programs now try to discourage. Modern Western civilization is the first one that offers no established popular bonding rituals, perhaps because most Christian doctrine is based on a deficient perception of human evolutionary nature.

The Vatican is a miniature America: everyone talks about sex, and yet all that talk intensifies the sexual borders between people until the body resembles a fort. Every day I heard of more officials who were eager to talk if their anonymity were guaranteed; I limited myself to Americans. Like most people, these priests were merely and bravely chasing after a combination of a good time and a higher purpose and meaning, mostly in splintered secret lives. Their faith was touchingly sincere, but their love for humanity seemed the result of a personal battle they daily carried out, less an impulse than a conscious denial of their repulsion and fear; more the mental exercise of an overextended willpower, like the self-control required to suppress the needs of their bodies, than a natural urge. The two seemed connected: every day a little more of our repression is visited on our hearts and bodies; when we hold to repression too long, we lose our innate compassion. I understand love as a spontaneous sweeping reaction to the world, like lust. Both can be at once ethereal and raucous, can cut through the ego's pretensions, reconnect us with the innocent joys of childhood, and feed our soul's hunger for ecstasy.

In the Vatican I understood that our organized religion asserts itself in our lives by the fundamental separation of sex from intimacy. Christianity influences the sex lives of millions, including those who are not religious. But none are more repressed and confused than the oppressors, the men of God, who struggle to live in both the old and the emerging moral order, and worry that they belong to neither.

"The truth shall set you free," Christ said.

Entering the Vatican can be a disorienting experience, like crossing the gates of the Parthenon only to discover it is still in use. Clattering along in my diminutive rental Fiat on winding cobblestone streets, past looming monasteries and hasty, trim men in flapping cassocks, I feel I've traveled into a monosexual medieval citadel. Fearful of losing an authority that extends far beyond its political borders, the Vatican stands frozen in time. The world's smallest sovereign nation, and only theocracy, is home to an efficient post office, a twenty-language radio and TV station, a publishing press, and two thousand bureaucrats whose prevailing task is to regulate the private lives of 900 million Catholics.

My personal task is to find out how these men—the supreme patriarchs, the chosen among the chosen—manage their own sexualities. As a woman, I am an anomaly here, hardly encouraged to intrude into this all-male professional club. But like 60 million American Catholics and many more millions of other Christians, I have long felt the Church's weighty restraining influence on my private life. Even as I pace these bumpy streets, I perceive the Vatican not as part of the city of Rome but an integral part of my visceral daily life. And I want to know how sexual repression affects those who serve it, and what they do about it.

For some eight hundred years, celibacy—the promise by priests and monastics to abstain from sex and marriage—has been a cornerstone of Church governance. St. Paul called celibacy "a gift from God." Ecclesiastical power and lawmaking is reserved for males who promise perfect and perpetual chastity.

The Vatican's high-powered, frustrated citizenry has only one sanctioned outlet: confession—a sacrament that teaches priests to keep the Church's secrets (as confessors) while keeping no secrets from the Church (as confessees). The compulsion to hide nothing from a system shrouded in sanctioned secrecy is the peculiar genius of the Catholic faith; guilt and denial bind its people together with sober intimate chains that unregulated sexuality could loosen. All the Vaticaners I meet open up to me with a willing childlike urgency that reflects this ingrained habit of cathartic verbal release.

The monsignor is one of the dignitaries in charge of "moral affairs in the Vatican." He likes vintage champagne and wild strawberries for lunch; and, like St. Jerome, who showily counseled and chastised aristocratic women, Monsignor likes to surround himself with attractive, rich, educated, or titled Catholic women on whom he bestows his friendship as a blessing.

One such radiant, devout American expatriate provides our introduction. Our lunch at her small sunny villa is refined, gracious. The gathered women fuss over their black-clad disheveled luminary. The air pulses with confused hormones, the birds chirp, huge flower arrangements scent the room. I realize the priesthood is designed for a life of uninterrupted courtship—an exciting showdown of desires and wills that never culminates and so never needs to end. It seems a pleasantly chivalric way to live, but juvenile.

Potbellied and exuberant, stooping with enviable unself-consciousness, communicating with twinkling beautiful Irish eyes and air-chopping gestures, Monsignor strikes me as the quintessential man of pleasure. So I ask him how, in a city where the most popular TV game show lets the players strip their clothes for points, can Vatican men stay sexually controlled. Unlike his native Boston, the Vatican is a Mediterranean culture. Isn't it harder to abstain where lust is omnipresent? Monsignor nods affably. His answer is not the coy denial I expect. "Roman culture," he agrees, "unlike the Anglo-Saxon, tolerates contradictions. It's taught me to accept my nature as well as my faith." The women listen in rapt silence. We're drinking antique Dom Pérignon and are served platefuls of heavenly pastas. Wild berries over homemade pear sorbet in ice sculptures and aged monastic port await for dessert.

Monsignor thinks it is time to bring priestly sexuality into the open. "Celibacy is discipline, not doctrine," he explains. "You don't *have* to believe in it to be Catholic. It's just one of the laws that run a large institution—an outdated mechanism of control. For centuries our priests married. Orthodox priests still do. For the last thirty years we've had married deacons and married converted Anglicans. It's common sense that lay people can use healthy, sexually functional role models. No one in the Church today cares about priestly marriage, but massive organizations take a long time to change. The Vatican recognized the earth is round just two years ago," he chuckles, clinking champagne glasses with us all.

"It *will* change in my lifetime," he adds, "but for now, we must respect celibacy." Does that mean that for now all priests are asexual? "No, the Church knows that we can't *not* be sexual, because we *are* sexual. Celibacy means no *marriage*. Chastity or continence means not having sex, and that's discipline for all Catholics." I bypass these preposterous fine points. So are you allowed to masturbate? I persist. "I would have thought as a feminist you wouldn't encourage that sort of thing," he taunts me. Masturbation is better than nothing, I argue. "It's nice to get the parameters right," he jokes on. The women moan and rearrange their taut bodies, utterly besides themselves with nervous discomfort. They're afraid for him. For themselves, they are afraid of facing his palpable maleness this openly.

To our hostess's unfeigned shock, I next ask him if he is a virgin. "I was three months from being married to this girl I loved for five years," he answers indirectly, always convivial. "I still love her. She's still not married. *She* gave me up. She's been living with a chap. I think she realized, even though I did not realize it then, that my heart wasn't entirely hers, because of this other *thing*—God. I hated her for it for a long time. I joined the clergy, and I've since learned to respect her enormously. I suspect that decision cost her her happiness. She'll go to heaven for that." I think: Religion *is* the ultimate justification. It has justified conquest and genocide, romantic failure and sexual rejection. It's historically common for a broken heart or sexual difficulty to lead a man to the priesthood, where life's parameters are safely narrow, and freedom of choice and personal responsibility are moot.

After coffee, the women tacitly kiss his ring and leave the two of us alone on the velvet couch. With only a few tangible inches and my tape recorder between us, Monsignor crosses his stout legs languorously and laughs brusquely, throwing his head back—a man at ease in his flesh. "One of my jobs is to be moral adviser to priests who fall in love," he volunteers. "Just because they fall in love, they don't need to leave the Church. Most priests *can* love the opposite sex without jumping into bed. And if there's no evil intent, a priest can even fall, pick up, and carry on. The problem is when, in the nuptial covenant with his people, a priest mixes his symbols and deceives himself into sexual rather than spiritual union, in his eagerness to show God's acceptance. A priest can easily elicit sexual responses in Church members, just as psychiatrists do in their patients. To take advantage of *that* is unethical."

He admits there are no official Vatican statistics on priestly sexuality. "Like there are no cases of pedophiliac priests in Italy that we know of," he explains. "Of course, there *must be*—it would be most *unnatural* if there weren't. But here they are not reported. I'd say thirty percent of local priests have mistresses. Italians don't care. They don't want their priests to seem unvirile, actually. This paranoia with sex is an Anglo-Saxon problem, very Protestant. Unlike older cultures that have learned to separate society from faith, America suffers from the contradictions between its amoral capitalism and its religious righteousness; for this reason it now clamors for moral reform. In Rome I live in my own flat; I have my [female] cousin stay with me a lot. Nobody cares. It's like the difference in the way I drive my car in the States and in Rome: here no one goes by the rules. No one has argued about contraception in Italy for thirty years. They use it; they clap for the Pope; they see no inconsistency. The Pope tries his best, but he knows life is complex and priests *are* lonely. When you are critically lonely, you look for solace—in drink, or woman, or now a man." I ask if in private the Pope condones the normal sexual failings he publicly condemns. Monsignor laughs again, apparently amused: "The Pope says: 'There's an awful lot under this big tent.' Outside the sexual bit, the Pope is very liberal. He laughs at the ironies of the Church. He has convinced people he's conservative because it makes him more effective. He knows the facts of human nature. But he fears that if you allow one thing, you'll lose hold of everything."

In fact, the Holy See, angered by his inability to control America's "endemic" scandals, has stonewalled the issue of priestly sex, even as polls confirm that half the American clergy (and 80 percent of young priests) favor the option to marry. As a result, while America's Catholic population has risen drastically since the sixties, the number of diocesan priests has fallen by 26 percent (it will be 40 percent by 2005) and of seminarians by 80 percent. More than a thousand American priests resign each year to get married; 10 percent of American priests leave the active priesthood within five years of ordination, and 25 percent within twenty-five years, most to marry. Tens of thousands more have applied to be released from their vows and spend years waiting for a response from the logjam of the papal bureaucracy. (Laicization can only be authorized by the Pope.) Today, the Association of Catholic Priests and Their Wives counts eighty thousand married priests—20 percent of the total active clergy—who stand ready to resume service. But because of the official apathy, most priests forfeit their vow of abstinence without leaving the Church in which they have invested their lives. Monsignor calls them "management problems."

I have been here a week and I am deeply surprised by how disenchanted Vatican insiders are with their own celibacy vows. Monsignor is not an exception. Papal infallibility notwithstanding, everyone I speak to claims that John Paul II's death will signal the end of proscribed celibacy. These priests don't think that "to be carnally minded is death" (Romans 8:5). Instead, they think that unreasonable bans on abortion, birth control, homosexuality, and women's ordination will be relaxed when priests openly join the rest of the human race in accepting the tribulations of our sexual imperative.

What they don't discuss is that, in practice, celibacy is already obsolete. Experts estimate that only 2 percent of Catholic priests sworn to perpetual celibacy achieve it.* At any given time, 20 percent are involved in sexual affairs with

*These statistics are culled from Catholic publications. They are based on research conducted by Catholic priests like Richard Sipe who work within the Church as its unofficial sexologists and sex therapists.

women, 6 percent are having sex with minors, 8 percent are experimenting sexually otherwise, and anywhere from 30 to 60 percent are actively or inactively homosexual. And 80 percent of those who practice celibacy masturbate occasionally. The carnal lives of the Church's self-chosen celibates are the ultimate proof of the dysfunction of its moral autocracy. From 1982 to 1992 four hundred American priests were publicly reported for molesting minors; thousands were reported for seducing adults. Given the chain of scandals exposed by the U.S. media in the past decade, the news has ceased to shock, confidence in the Church has declined, insubordination has increased. The Church insists on official cover-ups to save the social esteem of the priesthood. Because the Church uses its priests as moral examples to control the laity's libido, to acknowledge priestly sexuality would be to open the door to sexual anarchy. So the hierarchy still advocates a morality that dates back to St. Augustine, the libertine who converted to Christianity in the fourth century, and then eloquently equated sex with perdition; Augustine's pessimistic belief in the moral impotence of humans prevailed because it justified the need for universal papal domination.

Father John's students rave about his dedication, honesty, and genius. As a preeminent Latin scholar, John translates the Pope's writings and encyclicals into the official Latin. He is fluent in eight languages. He is also a black sheep who criticizes the Pope for "ruining Catholicism." Monsignor describes John as an iconoclast, the son of a poor Maine plumber who joined a monastery as a teen to escape a career in plumbing, and who now "lives in a bare cell alone with Cicero."

I am waiting for John to come out of his towering moldy monastery. I examine the stone walls, afraid of raising suspicions, until the massive metal gate is raised and a fit middle-aged man exits carrying an empty jug of wine he's just shared with his Latin class. He wears blue-jean shirt and pants from

JCPenney. "My uniform," he slurs. "When I wear it out, I buy a new one. After twenty-seven years, they still give me a hard time here about jeans. 'With the Pope down the hall from me,' I say, 'you have worse problems, so shut up!'"

At first, John is viciously aggressive. "What is your *problem?*" he keeps sneering about my desire to interview him. He has a beer gut, a ramshot spine, a proud strut. His half-shut eyes see the world with generic disdain. He's the fifty-year-old spitting image of a West Village queen: he roars in laughter, speaks in aphorisms, squints at passersby, and squeaks when excited. He's nothing if not provocative.

We sit at a dusty sidewalk table in the nearest trattoria, and after we get our drinks and he sufficiently intimidates me by bombarding me with personal questions, he takes off: "Augustine's word for the original sin is *concupiscentia*: lust for sex, power, possession—not sexual lust in isolation. Does the Pope stress that? No! Augustine says *empathy* is the antidote to greed. Does the Pope do that? He threatens. Augustine is blamed these days only because of the silence of most Christian writers in addressing sexuality." If the Church can revise its views on slavery and witchcraft, or repeal the Latin Mass and the mortal sin of eating meat on Friday, why can't it reexamine clerical (and secular) sexuality? "It's this terrible idea that we're special if we're celibate. I call it our Deformation. The Pope thinks he was chosen by God to bring unity to the Church, and he mistakes unity for iron-hand uniformity. But he grew up in Communism—Marxists are more repressed even than Catholics." He shouts and rages at me, the outsider, for forcing him to defend his Church, *and* rages at his Church for its inert rigidity, for carelessly "impeding human growth." He strikes me as a man of convictions, not fully aware of his emotions. "If there's not room for everyone in the Church," he says, "there is room for no one. The next Pope has to redefine our morality. They're afraid if you pull out one or two bricks, the whole edifice will fall! So it's falling already. The Scriptures don't talk about sex! The Church is teaching many things for which there is no foundation! *That* gets me. As for the value of our God-given *tradition*—hey, we were sure the earth was flat!"

He peppers this fevered speech with screechy gossip. He mentions a cardinal who is HIV-positive; brings up the Pope's youthful erotic verses; explains that Italian dioceses have special funds to support their priests' illegitimate children. He tells me stories about a priest who strangled his boyfriend, about a director of the Sistine choir who died in the arms of a prostitute, a tribunal priest arrested for exposing himself in a public park, a protest march in France by mistresses of priests, a bishop in Switzerland who announced he was to be a father and 75 percent of the public supported him even as the Pope defrocked him. In between these relished indiscretions, he makes the childish sign of sealing his lips. But he can't quench his semiecstatic urge to speak out.

"Modern Catholicism," he says, "does not enlighten. At best, it protects." From what? He ignores this, as he does all of my attempts to establish a reasonable flow of question and answer. "Priestly sex is the most serious crisis the Church has faced since the Reformation," he goes on. "Sex-related lawsuits have cost my Maine diocese $7 million. But I have sympathy for my 'affected' brethren: when I made my vows at sixteen, I didn't know what the hormones might do to me at sixty. I've had dozens of classmates who ran off to marry nuns late in life. I have ninety brothers in my monastery here. I see a lot. And in my room, I have no one to talk to." John's order takes a vow of silence; inside the monastery, no one chats.

I doggedly try to access his personal experience. Can priests help admiring pretty girls in the street as they would admire springtime blossoms, etc.? "For me, abstinence is freedom," he retorts, and I realize he is a virgin. "My sexuality is nongenital. I'm free to do what I want, admire what I want, *because* I take chastity for granted. Nothing can trap me. For me it solves problems—it's like these clothes. I know what I wear every day. I have perfect clarity. No sex means no complications, no ambivalence. I like not being attached. Sex is ownership: I don't want to possess a car or a house, so when I hear people talk this way ('I want him,' 'You're mine'), it's scary. But mine is not the typical Vatican way." I ask if some people may be genetically predisposed to chastity. "But you don't have to renounce sex to communicate with God!" he illogically fires back with his flair for argument. "Most people would say the opposite: an injection of sex might help you find God, considering the way we're genetically made." I now sense his sexual "freedom" has been obtained at immense sacrifice.

When we part, John calls after me in a shaky voice that echoes through the deflating purple Roman dusk: "Visit the Vatican; you'll see why Luther had an epileptic fit at St. Peter's!"

I've never been surrounded by such a relentless evocation of naked flesh as I see in the Vatican palace: every magnificent inch of ceiling, staircase, floor, and wall is an unapologetic display of homoerotic imperial art, an ostentatious hodgepodge fostering no conceivable intimacy with an immaterial, repressive God. At the other extreme of this decadent overstimulation is the accumulation of memento mori slogans (the "Remember Death" Catholic staple): Death—the great equalizer, the ultimate democrat—adds an ominous aspect to the lapis cherubs and gilt pineapples. An old priest next to me tells me the seventh floor of the Vatican's basement contains the largest collection of pornography in the world—including hundreds of drawings by Michelangelo, Caravaggio, and other masters that were acquired to prevent their general consumption. According to my source, the Vatican remains one of the biggest consumers of porn in the world for this reason.

I am on my way to the Vatican library to meet Mark, a married defrocked priest and counselor from Baltimore, but as I make my way from room to room through the dazed throng, I get so dizzy from the avalanche of color, curvature, texture, and epic musculature, of the unrequitable greed driving Popes to loot and hoard, that by the time I reach the library I feel nauseated, as if I'm suffering from the Stendhal syndrome ("dizziness and palpitations due to aesthetic overload," an illness first experienced by the French novelist in the local church of Santa Croce).

Mark is a balding, stocky, bearded Italian-American in a cheap suit, gold cross, and oversized glasses. I find him playing choral Mass on a computer. I need fresh air, so he takes me to a nearby reassuringly peaceful Trappist monastery that makes and sells "the world's best" eucalyptus liqueur and chocolate. As we sample them, he tells me this is the site of St. Paul's martyrdom: when his head was severed, it rebounded thrice, causing the three fountains we see to spring up. I say that every square inch of the Vatican hosts a macabre holy legend, but he cuts me off. "This is truth, not myth," he corrects me reverentially.

Mark and I end up in his rented marble-floored, squalid walk-up, where I meet his plain, soft-spoken wife, Laura, and share their antipasto and Chianti on their decrepit marble veranda. Laura is shy, subdued, wide-eyed. Mark is big, voluble, fervent. They tell me they met at church functions in New Jersey and, unexpectedly, fell in love. Their relationship stayed secret for three years. Mark had never seen a naked woman before. He told himself it was wrong, but it felt right. He didn't recognize himself. He contemplated suicide. He checked into a mental hospital. He cried after each time they had sex and promised never to touch her again. They devised schemes and bargains to keep him celibate—not drinking alcohol, staying outdoors, going only "so far"—until Mark would break his own abstinence with a flimsy excuse, and then blame Laura for letting him lapse. "Priests are blindly narcissistic," he says.

The affair was unworkable. Mark was a good priest who

loved his Church and hated cheating on her. But, sexually, he was a fourteen-year-old in a man's body: naive and desperate. Laura bore the burden of his guilt with patience. When her diaphragm failed, Mark refused to accept her pregnancy. He felt he was being punished for betraying his priesthood. Then he had a revelation: God had sent him a child as a message against sexual shame. He decided to marry Laura and join the crusade to end enforced celibacy. He says having a family made him complete: "I believe that in principle I am still a priest. I feel chaste. I think knowing a woman makes a man a wiser, more compassionate priest." Before he met Laura at the age of thirty-five, Mark had suffered from spontaneous emissions. He had never masturbated, yet he could sit in the library or his room and experience ejaculation with no physical movement; he had erections while saying Mass and even spontaneous ejaculations while consecrating the host. It had shamed and tormented him, for his conscious thoughts were always on his prayer. After meeting Laura, these accidents stopped. He now thinks they were an expression of his love of God. "A person's body and soul," he says, "do coincide."

Mark is in the Vatican researching the history of celibacy for a book he hopes to publish. He says St. Augustine did not advocate priestly celibacy any more than Christ or the Apostles; but he did pave the way by identifying sexual desire as proof of, and penalty for, the original sin. Whereas early Christians understood the tale of Adam and Eve as a lesson on free will and procreative responsibility (noting God's mandate that they name and populate the earth), Augustine read it as a tale of our carnal captivity transmitted through intercourse from generation to generation. And this is how arbitrary our sexual morality is. Even those of us who are not Christian or who treat the Bible as literature live by the edicts of a culture indelibly shaped by this one man's reading of a paragraph written down by Hebrew tribes thousands of years ago.

Clerical celibacy was not enforced until the eleventh century, during Pope Gregory VII's reforms. The Pope's primary objective was to stop priests' families from inheriting Church lands at a time when abbots and clerics were passing religious property to their sons and simony (the selling of ecclesiastical offices) was a bustling business. Mandatory celibacy also conferred an air of superiority on the clergy and helped consolidate the Pope's moral and geopolitical prestige.

The ironic result of sexual segregation, Mark says, is the tolerance of clerical homosexuality by the homophobic Church. "The seminaries desensitize us to the social norm and foster effeminacy, so men turn to each other for intimacy. This system produces the prissy gay bishops who recruit for priests in peep shows. I don't mind that gays don't 'transmit life.' I mind that they cultivate a politics of dishonesty in the Church. Unlike priests who wish to marry, homosexuals have no reason to leave the Church; there are more gays in the Church now than in the general population, and they are not accountable. I met a monk here who left the Church because his duties included procuring male whores for his monsignor. Eighty percent of sexually abusive priests were similarly abused at seminary. De Sade learned whipping and sodomy from his Jesuit teachers. Celibacy is our most serious disability. The Church won't even commission boards to monitor its priests, on the premise that God is our only judge. I call it our hypocrisy. I'm not allowed to officiate because I married, but I know a pastor who picks up truckers at diners, gets beaten up, and in the morning says Mass and confesses people. Any priest who keeps his sex life secret keeps the right to serve; and if he's reported, he's only recycled to a new diocese. Yet the Vatican will strip a theologian of his teaching license if he advocates optional celibacy, even if he lives a chaste life. The system is crumbling under its own corruption and duplicity. The Pope can't know these facts and not shudder."

I spend some days reading at the library, and this is what I learn: even the most cursory history of Christianity reveals that sexual repression is irrelevant to Christ and his vision of heaven on earth; it is relevant only to the historical ambitions of political and religious leaders. Until the late antique period Christians viewed the flesh of Christ as continuous with human flesh. That was the genius of the faith: in the conception, birth, and death of Christ, every human physiological process was reaffirmed. Christ's incarnation expunged the "disorder" introduced into the human body by Adam's fall; it was our allegoric victory over death. As Christianity came to dominance, it switched its emphasis away from life, toward the democracy of death. Synods and encyclicals transposed Christ's vision of a nonauthoritarian society onto the promised society of heaven, thereby justifying suffering in this world. Martyrdom became the mortar of the faith. Entry to that afterlife was kept in the hands of the hierarchy who bartered it at will and often for profit (selling indulgences to raise money for the Church was why purgatory was invented). Most of these distortions happened as the totality of the Jesus movement became infected by the Greco-Roman puritanism that espoused the dichotomy between body and soul, and by the Stoic and Essene ethic that reacted to Rome's degenerate mores by advocating a "boycott of the womb." As Christian leaders emulated pagan doomsday forebodings, Porphyry's phrase, "Shame at being in the body," came to represent Christian piety; Jesus' message of freedom came to mean "freedom *from* the body."

Before his conversion in the fourth century, Augustine had belonged to the Manichean sect, which practiced continence and saw the sexual instinct not as the merciful gift from God that helped Adam overcome death, but as a demonic possession of the world, a permanent evil present in all humans, a token of mindless bondage to the animal cycle of mortality. Anxious to make himself a place in his new faith, and to expiate his guilt for keeping a longtime mistress, fathering a son with her, and banishing her for a society wife, Augustine passed these old-world fatalisms into Christian society by defining sexual drive as *poena reciproca*, a punishment on Adam's descendants. Augustine's theology was predicated on one line from Genesis: "And the eyes of both of them were opened and they knew they were naked." He narrowed theology to the paradigm of the "indecent" *summa voluptas* of orgasm, which escaped the limits of the conscious self that knows and obeys God. He theorized that sexual pleasure infected the conceived child with eternal damnation: sex and the grave stood at each end of every human life and between them roared a cascade of misery, ignorance, malice, and violence. His symbiosis of sex and perdition fortified the celibate clerical state. Many learned bishops and monks challenged his reading, but they were denounced as heretics. Disobedience became the cause of all evil, and sex its manifestation. Christians who disagreed were excommunicated, tortured, burned, sent on far-flung penances, or imprisoned. Theologians went so far as to preach that "isolation from sex" was a reason Christ had come to earth.

The real reason Christians came to live in fear, just as they had in Roman and Pharisaic times, was the Church's other deviation from Christ's radically egalitarian teachings: the creation of a monarchic bishop system and all-male priesthood. The first step toward this despotism was the establishment of a permanent priesthood that acquired disciplinary powers and took over the duties, tiaras, and pomp of emperors. The second step was the declaration of the primacy of the Roman bishop, who replaced the collective bishops as the supreme head of the Church. The final step was papal infallibility, proclaimed in 1870 with the stroke of a threatened Pope's pen, that effectively turned the Vatican prelate into God.

Thin, neat, reticent, Father Matthew is a thirty-eight-year-old gay sex addict based in Denver, Colorado. He is a highly educated priest slated to become president of a major American Catholic university. He is also a regular at the seedy meat racks of every European capital; he takes DepoProvera (a female contraceptive used as a sexual appetite suppressant), receives psychiatric therapy, and seasons his staid discourse with infantile recovery-speak such as "stinking thinking" and "attitude of gratitude." He pronounces his words guardedly, as if they were exotic and potentially explosive oblations.

Monsignor thinks Matthew should leave the Church before he becomes a litigation risk: "If he can't rid himself of the addiction, he should rid himself of his celibacy vows," he tells me. "His faith can't help him. Ecclesiastic therapists call it 'the celibate psychosis.' As I understand, homosexuals can't help being sick. He takes a wonder drug, he goes to Gay Anonymous; he picks up men there, too. For the sake of an orgasm, he'll risk arrest, assault, VD, public shame, his career. All we can do is advise him and pray the vice squad won't pick him up for soliciting. And he looks like a wimp to me—not a man I'd play rugby with." Nevertheless, Matthew has such a God-given talent for fund-raising that the Pope knows him by name.

I never learn Matthew's real name. We meet clandestinely in a posh suburban restaurant near the catacombs. He is tan and stylish in sandy silk turtleneck, linen blazer and pants; his hair is waxed, his shoes spit-polished, his voice scoldingly exhausted, his body language so comatose that I can't imagine him lustful. Does he practice safe sex? I ask. "AIDS would be the end of my addiction and the start of my martyrdom," he replies, forcefully and surprisingly, exposing the extent of his devastation. "Priests with AIDS are well cared for. They're 'out,' accepted. I'm more tortured now. I literally can't trust myself." He holds a Marlboro between two long fingers that come between me and his face like a defensive veil, and with each puff he regains his unexpressive composure.

It seems to me self-defeating to isolate his sexual behavior and regard it as separate from the rest of him, I say. Many of us feel some shame about our sexuality, but we try to overcome it. If we embrace the Catholic paradigm that sex is a sickness, we'll inevitably experience our primal urges as a psychotic disorder rather than a natural need. Isn't it an act of hubris to believe that we can control or even fathom human instinct? To me, desire is what makes the world go round.

Matthew says it's too late for him: he learned that sex is a pathology at a very early age; his brain is "programmed to read the effect of those natural opioids on the medial forebrain bundle as negative. Drugs like Prozac alter the levels of these signals but not their interpretation." If sex weren't such a difficult area for the Church, I say, there might be no demoralized priests. The general view in our culture is that chemical imbalance *causes* psychological compulsions, but as Dr. Avram Goldstein, a pioneer in the area, has written, "in the final analysis psychology *is* biology," which means that our cultural values determine our biological responses. Matthew's guilt is compounded by the Christian teaching that one's sexual behavior is under one's control. Unlike laic addicts who get drawn into compromising affairs, Matthew sees his hankering for any physical intimacy as a de facto spiritual failing. "I never stop fighting it. I live like St. Anthony in the desert." But doesn't he think sexual pleasure *can* be ethical, even holy? "Not in my lifetime," he responds. So what's the penalty for violating his vows? "None. Unless you count eternal hellfire." I ask if he believes in hell. "Yes," he replies matter-of-factly. This sounds incongruous coming from a man who believes in brain neurotransmitters. Does he hold the Devil accountable for his condition? "Sometimes metaphorically. Most of the time quite literally," he mutters. "Many here believe that the Devil is just persecuting the Church in this prurient way." That ignores personal responsibility, I protest. "Oh, free will; but that's why Catholicism has been a successful religion for so long," he tells me.

He claims the homosexual contingent in the Vatican is huge. "This is the best hiding place," he says. I ask why he doesn't leave the Church. "Because I am a good priest," he says. "The Church is losing too many valuable priests as it is. I wanted to see you," he continues, "to tell you how upsetting it is to people like me that sexuality is at the forefront of our ecclesiastical discussion. Even in this bloodiest century in human history, Catholic doctrine views humanity's crimes as being committed in the bedroom. Carnal sin has superseded all sins because the Church knows that if it can control the innermost desires of kings and plebes alike, if it can persuade people not to be sexual, there's nothing it can't control. But the emphasis on sex obscures larger sins, like usury, which is the basis of our capitalist system and has made us debt slaves with credit cards, mortgages, deficits. There are many grave sins we overlook because sex throws petty sand in our eyes and distracts us. The poor get poorer, the rich richer, nuclear arsenals get larger, the planet gets more destroyed and overpopulated. I believe in the salvation of every soul. Even at gay bars, I preach to clients. Catholic means *everyone*. I believe in the sanctity of the Pope, his *being* the Church. I am bound to obey him. But this has to be the last Pope of his kind."

The Christ of the New Testament is irrepressibly inclusive and physical, fearlessly attuned to reality. He saw the spirit as inextricably joined with the body. He made his teaching physical. He whipped, groaned, kissed. He broke the Levitical taboos of cleanliness and purity that regulated dealings among people: he touched the blind, the dead, the lepers, the whores, the bleeding women, the forbidden castes. He put his trust in body language, invited intimacy, used his spittle to heal.

In his farewell meal, he showed that body and soul are one when he incited us to partake of his being. "Take and eat, this is my body which is given for you." As St. Thomas observes, Christ didn't say, "This bread is my body," but, "This is my body," indicating that "this" is bread no longer—it is his *flesh*. There is nothing puritanical in this rite of ingestion. Its vocabulary is sexual. It is Christ making love to us. Inside his bride Church, he is incarnate Presence. By swallowing the Eucharist we become united with the mystery of the material elements and resurrected through it: "Whoever eats my flesh and drinks my blood has eternal life, and I will raise him up" (John 6:54). This daily hallowed feast evokes our universal essential bond to the physical world, reminding us that we emerge from nature and return to it and for the short time when we remain a part of nature, we sustain our life by assimilating it into ourselves. "Take this . . . and drink from it: this is the cup of my blood." In its essence, Christianity is hedonic; its priests lead our communion with the ineffable mysteries of nature.

So it is shocking how soon after his deification the body-restraining taboos Christ abhorred were reinstated by his Church. As Jesus the iconoclast was turned into Jesus the icon, his Church became the new (paralyzed) body of Christ. The Gospels give less attention to his martyrdom than to his miracles, but his Church capitalized on the goriness of his crucifixion to hold us in fear of all physical being through centuries of worshiping the aesthetic of suffering. The sexual body became so taboo that, even in our post-Freudian world, we dread the deranging effects of lust and seek our pleasure in secret, associating bodily desire with transgression. But the distinctive feature of Christianity remains that our God was embodied, in order to confirm and heal our bodily nature. Unlike Zeus or Yahweh, Christ was human, birth to death. God's becoming flesh is the greatest scandal in human history.

Luke is a Franciscan instructor of Bible semiotics at the Angelico University. He was born in Atlanta and his mother wanted him to be a priest. He has scrubbed, angular looks; high, pale cheekbones; a nervous shyness around the lips. We meet at the idyllic courtyard of his monastery, populated by laurel-wreathed statues of monks. What persuades a young man in the late twentieth century to lock himself up for six abstinent years to study theology? I ask. He mentions the passions of saints, writhing Pentecostals, Christian erotic psalms, "all the fun of sublimation." He ends up quoting Kant and Hegel, and, as he proceeds from thesis to antithesis, he is moved to illustrate his point with a Schubert sonata. All of a sudden, I find myself being hushedly rushed into the sanctum; I follow him up creaky oak stairs, and into an old white cell, quiet as a crypt, adorned only with a metal cross and a portrait of the founder of the order. I get seated on a tattered armchair across from this monk's carefully made narrow bed, as if it were the most natural thing in the world.

Luke clicks off the Mac on his rickety desk, puts on the CD, procures cheap wine from a mini fridge. We listen, sip, and nod until the bottle is empty. He recites poems. He mentions a friend who tried to kill himself in his cell last week. As the alcohol saturates my empty stomach, I shut my eyes momentarily. All at once, his tongue lands in my mouth. He is staring at me with a vigilant expression that seems to be preparing for the best and the worst, fearing both. His kiss is expert. His body is not touching mine. My mind races to stories not of sexually active seminarians, but of the dozens of priests facing public exposure of their sexual activity who commit suicide in America every year. To protect us both, I pull away and say, "I thought priests couldn't do that."

In a whirlwind, he apologizes profusely ("I've never reached orgasm," he insists; "it's a matter of pride to me"), already looking ahead to his absolution with the self-immolated gaze of a binger craving a purge. He gathers my belongings and sneaks me out. Midnight hour has struck and no visitors are allowed in the Vatican cloister, least of all a woman; so I crouch below the dashboard of his Fiat until we pass the Swiss Guards flanking the city gates in their puffy, Michelangelo-designed, colorful uniforms.

After we cross the Tiber, I ask if he resents his celibacy. "It's a fact," he says, looking at the empty road straight ahead, "like the sun rising east. I fall in love, but I love God more; in the end, I'd rather be the beloved than the lover." But sex is a divine unmasking, I say, a type of communion. I say more: Sexuality is an instinct as primal as, and complementary to, religion. Our holy rites are essentially meant to ensure fertility. Fighting nature is a product of human vanity, not of divine injunction. To me, any systematic demonization of the flesh is antilife and anti-Christ, a dangerous form of atrophy. Besides, at any moment, a natural disaster could send us back to the caves where we started, fornicating vehemently for our survival; then all our conceited moralizing about who's allowed to lie with whom, when, and how would be revealed for the absurdity it is.

Luke returns that the Pope recommends abstinence even for married couples as a source of peace and bliss. I protest that, in real life, most people use sex to express love and to feel bliss. Luke reads me the litany of rules: Every sexual act between spouses outside the purpose of procreation is a venal sin. Every sexual thought, word, desire, and action outside marriage is a mortal sin. But this, I point out, lumps as equal transgressions having a wet dream and taking hundreds of pictures of nude girls, or oral sex and bestiality. No wonder priests are confused. Luke steals a glance at me and goes on: Lustfully exciting a spouse is a mortal sin. Coitus interruptus, masturbation, nighttime ejaculation—any squandering of semen—are "very grave" sins. So, like a pornographer, I say, the Pope defines sex as degradation. Luke is looking scared.

I can't sleep that night. I worry about harming the men I've spoken to. Then I decide that the Church is bound to honor the human body. The Incarnation and Resurrection of Jesus are affirmations of the body. Christ teaches us not pain but transformation. I pray his Church can find the courage to transform itself and transcend its legacy. Until then, the Christian martyrs of our day will be men like Matthew and Luke, or Fathers Gauthe and Fontenot of Lafayette, Illinois, who molested one hundred to two hundred boys each: *they* are the lost souls, sociopathic sacrifices to the Catholic cause of sexual control.

In the end, money may be the driving factor for moral reform: America's $500 million in official losses from child molestation lawsuits alone is six times the Vatican deficit; this doesn't count the costs for the rehabilitation of convicted priests, the transfers of accused priests, dispensations of harassed minors, men and women, sex therapy costs for the clergy, and so on. Thousands of cases of sexual abuse by priests are still pending in American courts. At any one time (since 1989) three dozen priests are incarcerated for sexual crimes. Victims of Clergy Abuse (LINKUP) held their first national meeting in October 1992. Local officials assure me the Vatican will bend in the face of this monstrous financial reality because "ultimately it is a bureaucracy, and what greases its wheel is ambition, backstabbing, and budgetary needs." They may as well be discussing the U.S. military, not a spiritual fraternity. "The Vatican," they joke, "is the city with the most faith in the world—because so many priests lose their faith here."

The next day I run into Monsignor in his black mufti buying the *New York Times* by the Pantheon. He shakes my hand warmly and says, a kind smile lighting up his sensual face, "You met Luke." Flabbergasted, I quickly slip into the indigenous secrecy and shame; I mutter ignorance. I'm fighting a dismal sensation of moving underwater. "He couldn't help himself; you moved him," he adds. Monsignor's brotherly instinct is to shield his priest, so he remakes Luke into the ingenue led astray by my practiced charms. And I say nothing. I feel guilty. I realize this is why so few sexual victims of priests speak up; this is how otherwise decent, popular priests can run adolescent sex rings and convince themselves they're not being sexual. We are all morality eunuchs.

Los Angeles:
Tales from the Crypt

"I will be a bridegroom in my death, and run into't as to a
   lover's bed."

Shakespeare, Antony and Cleopatra

Within the schism that separates spiritus *from* corpus, *and so
frustrates the quest for wholeness in a human being, nothing
became plainer to me in my travels than the conscious struggle
of most of my subjects for a modicum of integration. They often
didn't understand why they felt dead inside so much of the time,
why they lived in ways they didn't particularly enjoy; I could see
it was not their lack of imagination that caused their distress,
but the strictures they had accepted as the time-proven bounds of
life. If they were divided between those who possess too little
imagination and those who possess too much, they nonetheless
met on the same battlefield where the nature clashed with culture. "Hell," wrote Sartre, "is other people." And was it not the
respect and love of others that so often kept my interviewees hidden from the scrutiny of daylight? Between the brute needs of
some and the idealized hopes of others, the growing numbers of
marginalized Dickensian subcultures I gained entry into, began
to startle more than bewilder me. Was a large enough quantitative shift in our sexual urges sufficient to create a qualitative
one? And where, if qualitative, would the revolution end?*

In a society devoted to public scavenging and condemnation of private behavior, how could any of the people who wrestled sexual demons hope to achieve the desired union of mind and body without risking the lives that, on the surface, they lived? To what extreme would some need to go?

The neighborhood is orderly, well-maintained, and unscarred, a familiar testimony to human zeal and prerogative. The land is arid and uneven, but no one remembers that. Every home has a flat verdant lawn, a finical flower bed, a double garage. Nothing extraneous or accidental meets the eye. The house I am looking for is decorated by granite slabs and a Lilliputian pebbly moat. It is the picture of a curbed masculinity, the work of a man anxious to convince himself there are still ruthless elements to be tamed outside his abode. The sprawling interior is replete with floral cloth wreaths, potted plants, lace doilies, family photos, and all the Rockwellian refuse with which people surround themselves to avoid facing the daily vacuity. Screechy voices lead me to the kitchen where Rob, his wife, Ruth, and their two young girls are having breakfast. Rob is busy feeding himself eggs and bacon, and Ruth has a shouting girl perched on each thigh and is sticking creamy spoonfuls into their mouths while they emit rapid-fire irrational questions. Rob pours me a Mickey Mouse cup of grape juice and gives me a flustered detailed update on the girls' health.

"Rob is a bully," I had been told by the couple who sent me to him. "Rob is unbelievably arrogant. He's an overwhelming man, a Jekyll-and-Hyde; he'll be sweet to you and stab you in the back." "Rob feels free to act without repercussion. If he's mean to you, call us," they warned. They were his confidants and fellow conspirators in the illegal sex sport whose enjoyment bonded them with indelible chains of friendship, so I believed, as I drove to his suburb, that I had reason to worry.

But I instantly find Rob frictionless and reliable. He isn't prickly or hiply ironic, and his smugness is harmless: he seems a boisterous man-child, bossy and needy, trapped in a life of rearing babies and bearing L.A.'s gridlock traffic. He wants to move to the open country, but there is a glitch: he is a part-time necrophiliac. Men can be lynched for smaller flaws in a small town, and corpses are scarce.

Rob's proclivity has been kept a secret from his family and colleagues since his early teens, when he was introduced to the freedom of being alone with a dead human in the funeral home of his best friend's father. His friend's family had owned the business for generations, and all the siblings worked in it. Rob wanted to work there summers, but his dad, a despotic real estate developer, forbade it. He visited it after hours with his friend. They were drawn there by a youthful morbid curiosity, a fascination with death, and eventually the desire to look up women's skirts and discover the secrets of female anatomy. They went as far as fingering female corpses in the erogenous zones and jacking off. They mostly derided the dead to show off their fearlessness, and bragged about it at school. Then they started going out with girls who let them make out, and their "pranks" were forgotten.

He is a giant of a man, bug-eyed, rufous-faced, bull-necked. He's packed in his stiff jeans airlessly, hunched and feral, and carries his colossal body as a burdensome accessory, like a war veteran. Rob is a product of domestic violence. He laughingly describes a time last year when his dad beat him and he curved into a fetal ball. As a teen, he internalized the pain as a mantle of machismo and went on a rampage of physical self-abuse. He spent his youth lifting weights and chasing brawls, punching and getting punched and leaving men for dead. As Dad took out his social frustrations on his son, Rob took his out on strangers. "My dad was tough and commanded respect; he had cause when he fought and I didn't. He had the substance, I had the act."

Having embraced the model of violence, Rob extended it to his sex life. He fucked in the style he rode dirt bikes or speedboats, fast and recklessly, without condoms, courting punishment "on a death course" fueled by coke, steroids, booze. "I went through a hundred women. Girls were sex tools, like rubbers a guy got rid of after sex, a dime a dozen." He called them "tear-offs" after the protective eye strips in motorcycle racing that racers tear off and throw away once they go through mud to have clear vision for their jump. He slept with "an Asian, a Mexican, a *Vogue* model who was a dumb stump but in bed she'd do anything, and four coeds at once." He had a goal to screw his way down the alphabet, from A (Annie, Bonnie, Cindy) to Z. His thrill came from the power of "making the sale." His favorite sex involved putting a girlfriend in a bathtub filled with ice cubes and leaving her there until she was cold and ashen enough to look dead; then he would lift her out and penetrate her.

We're on his living room couch. "Ruth was never a kicker and screamer," he adds, "but you don't marry the girl who sat on you while driving home from a rugby game, you marry the quiet clingy one. A couple needs opposites." Ruth has an open, strong-boned face and a modest, easygoing manner. His dad introduced them. They had a $60,000, three-hundred-people wedding, and months later a daughter. "Her Jewish mother taught her her tool is there to catch a man and breed, and then it isn't needed," Rob gripes. "We have sex twice a month. I don't want to hurt the mother of my girls, but she doesn't try. I buy her lingerie she hides. I got her a vibrator and nothing would make me happier than to think of her using it when I'm not here, but it sits new. When she's under construction, I'm deprived." He hopes she'll warm to it again after the girls grow up. "Most men I know are unfaithful because, after motherhood, women are not interested in sex. Men are dogs," he chuckles. "I have a throbbing woody in my pants all day. I like to do it twice a day. And I won't be reduced to using artificial vaginas."

I'm worried about offending Ruth, who keeps passing by as he talks, jauntily prancing from room to room, periodically calling out a seconding "Yeah" to his monologue, or mumbling, "Oh, honey," when he makes a crack about sex; but Ruth, I'm reassured, does what Rob says. "Ruth doesn't say anything, she trusts me, she doesn't count." "She never wants anything." "She doesn't have an opinion." She might as well be dead. "I'm the luckiest man," he brags, nibbling on an unlit cigar. Then he helplessly grabs his crotch.

Rob resumed his teenage experiments after his second daughter was born, three years into his marriage. His old school friend was still in the embalming business, and during a drunken stroll down memory lane, they revisited the "shop." The visits became a guys'-night-out ritual, and now Rob spends his Saturday nights with the boys at the mortuary. They tell the wives they're playing poker. Rob likes the camaraderie among morticians—"like a secret society," he says. "A hell of a lot of people would be into this if they had easy, private access to fresh bodies. I suspect half the people who come in contact with corpses play with them. They're hard not to take advantage of, lying there passive—you can act out any fantasy with them, you have access to the most taboo places and notions."

Early on, Rob had an extramarital affair and, though Ruth never knew, it devastated him. "I'd lie next to her at night feeling guilty in my own home. I learned my values. I still think about it all the time, but I don't act on it. That's why I think, in my heart, that I'm doing the right thing." In Rob's mind, necrosex hurts no one: he's not cheating on his wife with another woman and he isn't running the risk of falling in love and upsetting the balance of his life. "Necroplay requires only one consenting adult," he says. "The dead are dead, it's no harm to them; it is safe, painless sex. We use condoms," he assures me. "We probe and talk up a stream, or maybe take a different orifice each and really ham it up. If we're really hard up or had enough beers, we'll experiment with males, too. We don't score every week, but it's always a hoot. It's like entering another world. You leave your worries behind. You feel free."

How would he feel, I ask, if his own relatives were violated? "I don't care what happens to me after I go," he says confidently. "If I get felt up by a woman when I'm a stiff, what better way to end it all? Nelson Rockefeller died in flagrante with a young mistress. Now that's a happy ending. I guess I'd mind if it were my mom, but we never touch old people. We are normal." His reply sheds a stark, noxious light on a fantasy many people have: to die in a peak of sex.

Rob and I go for a stroll in a nearby grove. He limps and picks succulent oranges that I peel and eat, juices dripping through my fingers to my elbows, as we sit on the bristly dirt road looking out at smog-blurry mountains. A fine dust hangs in the air and coats everything. It smells of citrus blossoms and mud. I feel vigorously alive. He wonders how much anyone can control in life. As he talks, in his unviolent and pained voice, air explodes vehemently through his nose as if he were landed a blow. His hands reach out, but he restrains them from touching me. As his reservoir of secrets floods on, I suddenly and inexorably wonder if he'd like me better dead.

In "Sexual Attraction to Corpses: A Psychiatric Review of Necrophilia," Drs. J. P. Rosman and P. J. Resnick reviewed 122 cases of necrophilia. Like most therapists, they believe people are sexually hard-wired at an early age and can either deny or gratify their nature. They distinguished "genuine necrophilia" from "pseudonecrophilia" and classified the former into three types: necrophilic homicide, regular necrophilia, and necrophilic fantasy. They found that psychosis, mental retardation, or sadism are not inherent in necrophilic "disorder." The most common motive is the possession of an unresisting and unrejecting partner. Most necrophiles choose occupations that put them in contact with corpses or, conversely, discover their proclivity by having proximity to corpses.

The best-known contemporary necrophile is Karen Greenlee, who made national headlines in 1993 when she drove off in a hearse and, instead of delivering the body to the cemetery, vanished for days. The police found her in another county, overdosed on codeine Tylenol, and charged her with interfering with a burial. (Like most states, California has no law against necrophilia.) In the casket, next to the raped corpse, she'd left a long letter confessing to amorous episodes with forty dead men. The letter was full of remorse: "Why do I do it? Why? Fear of love, relationships. No romance ever hurt like this. It's the pits. I'm a morgue rat. This is my rat-hole, perhaps my grave." She got eleven days in jail for stealing the body, a $255 fine, and was placed on probation and medical treatment. The mother of the dead man sued for $1 million and settled for $117,000 in punitive damages. Greenlee admitted she had been breaking into funeral homes for years, and had been caught in the act and allowed to run away because funeral businesses are loath to report violations for fear of losing business. She had also attended the funerals of the men she molested, pretending to be an estranged girlfriend, and had sometimes broken into their fresh tombs.

She said she had been attracted to it all her life. As a child, she looked for excuses to wander about the neighborhood mortuary. As a college student, she worked in morgues. But after her arrest, as her notoriety grew, she became more comfortable with her sexuality, even proud of it. "When I wrote that letter, I was still listening to society," she said in an interview in 1998. "But the more they tried to convince me I was crazy, the more sure of my desires I became." She is now thirty-five, a pale, chubby "Goth chick," working on a novel in the style of 1997's

Exquisite Corpse by Poppy Z. Brite, and known in San Francisco for having "played with the dead." She lives on welfare, which she receives for being mentally unstable, and sleeps with men who see her necrophilia as a sign that she wasn't adequately pleased by the living. She claims that necrophilia is more prevalent than records show, and that the only thing that stops her from it these days is fear of AIDS, which is the main cause of death among the "group" she finds attractive—"men in their twenties."

The cultish attention Greenlee has received is indicative of a larger shift in the public's attitudes toward necrophilia. There are growing numbers of pseudonecrophiles—people who have no contact with the dead but like snuff and necroporn, act out necrophilic fantasies with their mates, talk dirty about corpses on the Net, or are aroused by images of slaughter and war lore. Groups like Leilah Wendell's American Association of Necrophilic Research and Enlightenment are sprouting, with the aim to bring like-minded necrophiles in touch, disseminate information about safe play, and fight discrimination. Offenders like Greenlee are admired by teens looking for new modes of rebellion. Mortuary science is gaining popularity as an exotic trade. And many people I asked told me they'd try necrophilia once, given a safe and reasonable opportunity, for instance with a just departed lover.

Courtney Heinz is a small thin blonde I sit next to at the bar of a Greek restaurant. She is reading *Child of God* by Cormac McCarthy, so I say I like the book. Her pale eyes brighten. The novel tells the story of a man in the hills of Kentucky who kills girls and has sex with them and decorates his fireplace with their hair. I mention to Courtney that I am in town to interview necrophiliacs. Her eyes bore into me suspiciously, then she asks me what I have learned. An hour later, she has tears in those eyes, and invites me to her home where we can talk.

We walk to her studio apartment in Hollywood, which

brims with velvet drapes, walls of old books, tall dripping tapers and vigil lights, feathers, beads and bottles of oils, kitsch necrophilic drawings, cat hair, dust, and tacky satanic adornments. She offers me "Sereni-tea" and puffed *mochi* cakes. She is twenty-eight, wears only black, has a Ph.D. in sociology and a mortuary science degree. She has never had intercourse with a living person. She describes herself as "a true romantic, one of the last ones left," a naturalist, and a Luddite.

"The dead are so lonely," she says. "The farewell touch from the living is the most important ritual for the dead. It's honoring the life they had." It's an old tradition, I say: the preparation of the dead for the voyage to the underworld has been observed fanatically by most cultures. Assuring our dead a safe passage to Hades or its equivalent and a comfortable afterlife is paramount to our peace of mind. The reason we've always, in one aspect or another, in the form of a pharaoh or our ancestors or the pietà, worshiped the dead is that they have access to the knowledge we most ardently covet: the secrets of death. Their inscrutable insight makes them into fetishistic objects. It's not much of a leap from that to see them as objects of desire, Courtney mordantly adds.

"I'm a recluse," she explains. "I find most people exhausting and ultimately crazy. Necrophilia isn't confusing. There are no mind games, no rejection, no funny looks, no long-term financial and emotional investment. It's like taking Communion." From early childhood, Courtney was obsessed with death. She collected dead birds, rats, roadkill, and buried them in a ritual that involved rubbing her body with the dead in "anointment." "When life turns into death, that crossroads is the most magical space to be in. It's shamanistic. Being alone with a corpse is a spiritual union for me, and every corpse is different. I don't mean just that it's a great anatomy lesson. They all teach me different things: they have their wisdom, innocence, memories, pain to impart. They teach me to perform on a healthier, more open sense of time, they teach me perspective. I don't live with the illusions of immortality most people harbor out there. And I'm in charge of my sexuality."

It strikes me as skin-crawling sex, I say. I can't imagine feeling sexual with a body that has no reaction to my passion, whose eyes register no rictus of lust and abandon, and where my desire exists as an absence. "Mechanically, it's not different," she objects. "What attracts me is the erection. Sudden death is erotic. When they hanged people in public, they used trap doors to hide the hard-ons of the dying men. The testicles of the dead swell to the size of cantaloupes. So you can keep your eyes on the genitals, and use them like dildos. I don't, because for me the *idea* of what I'm doing is what brings my release." I realize her sexuality is completely theoretical.

Courtney comes from a large wine-making family. She grew up outdoors, went to U.C. Davis, and wrote her dissertation on death. The day after her graduation, instead of taking a college teaching job, she walked into the town morgue and asked for work. At first she thought she wanted to write a book about the experience, but she soon decided the experience itself was her goal—it fulfilled her. She has never bothered having a social life; she "can't stand the blah-blah-blah."

After six months at the morgue, she'd seen five hundred autopsies. "You're freaked out for about a week," she explains. "You open a drawer and there are pairs of hands and buckets of brains. You can't get over the fact that these people were alive hours ago, like you are; it seems horrific. But you get used to it and come to see them like mannequins. You make jokes about them and nickname them, you cut them open, weigh their parts, boil the ribs, sever the head, then eat lunch. The guys I work with always comment on the bodies' penises or breasts, as if they were looking through a porn magazine— like, 'Those are some knockers.' That's considered normal. Every morning they walk in, look up the corpses' ages, and check out the nineteen-year-olds." There were two categories of bodies in the morgue: the memorable ones—people who jumped off buildings and shattered their bones, burn victims, bodies that floated in the bay for weeks, prostitutes found in garment bags in car trunks, people who cut their wrists, then took barbiturates, then drank Drano, then stabbed themselves. "The mess that came out of their bowels was intolerable. They can't be eroticized. Those who can be are heart attacks during sex, drug overdoses, men who accidentally strangulated themselves trying to achieve heightened orgasms. The first bodies I touched intimately were car crash victims that were pronounced dead on the scene—they were still warm, you could smell the alcohol in their blood. I realized these were human." Whereas Rob found dead bodies erotic because they are so easy to objectify, a bit like artificial vaginas, Courtney (like Greenlee) avoided the objectification inherent in her job by eroticizing her autopsies. "Then one day a boss said, 'Someone's been messing with this body. It looks like they were trying to fuck it,' and the idea was planted in my head. When I first kissed a cadaver, I imagined we were immortal. It's not the mute powerlessness and vulnerability that makes the dead sexy. It's what you can project on them. Their physical being is like a free empty canvas. You can imagine their past, their last desires. Once your senses get used to it, get less acute, your mind flies. It's the freedom that's sexy, not the transgression."

Isn't she afraid of getting caught? "Not really. I'm gentle. I leave no traces. I don't do violent penetration. I stimulate my clit with them, do sixty-nine, hold them. The body lying there makes me happy. The cold, the smell of death, the funereal aura excite me wildly." Has she tried to "cure" herself? "I went through all the private hell," she says, "wishing I were normal. I finally accepted myself. This is me, I might as well enjoy it. I'm miserable when I try to be what I am not. This is my calling. My family is uncomfortable with my strangeness. My older sister stopped talking to me. As far as she's concerned, I'm dead. My mother is supportive; she pays for my shrink. I made them all watch the film *Kissed,* and it's the first thing that has made a difference in my favor. People trust movies more than people." Courtney reminds me of the heroine of that film: both are possessed by the grave humorlessness of death-cult priestesses and holy virgins; and though their acts are depraved, they see them as sacraments. She says she feels pity for the dead bodies in her care: "I don't see my sexuality as a violation of the dead; I see it as a gift to them. Because we value longevity and health so much, the dead are untouchable in our society, like lepers. We're afraid to associate with them because we're afraid their death will rub off on us. It's superstition. I feel my life confirmed when I kiss a dead man, I feel strengthened by our contact, because I can do something most people fear. I'm helping the dead cross over more happily: my joy gives their spirits the final peace they need. My sexuality is our transcendence. And I don't find them ugly or gross. I don't treat them like spooks, but like humans. I make love to them. Sometimes, if I get passionate on top, the body purges blood from its mouth. But I see all death as another state of being. The problem is that our society doesn't have any cathartic mourning rites. We cover the dead with paint, so we won't have to face their reality, and get rid of them."

Jason is a mortician in a posh Rodeo Drive address, a darkly freckled workaholic who has built a lucrative career sticking his hands into the disintegrating orifices of dead people. He calls himself a makeup artist. He used to work with runway beauty-makers, painting the faces of famous nubile models, before he graduated to painting the faces of the dead. He lets me into his lair one balmy night, after everyone but the guard has gone home, so I can watch him work overtime. It is my unglorifiable version of a visit to the underworld—the forbidden trip that made Orpheus and Odysseus into legends; only

I'm down here to commune not with the spirits of the dead but their bodies.

I feel underdressed entering the immaculate part-private-chapel, part-corporate-boardroom funeral parlor. I recognize I am meant to feel intimidated and small and mortified. The reception hall is clean, stately, all polished brass and laquered wood. The juxtaposition of grand illusion and bottom-line reality, the combination of greed at the expense of doom and ostentation in the service of demise, give me pause; I feel like grieving. I resist the temptation to sit and contemplate the biggest questions of life. The overwhelming silence is deceptive: in the empty offices, phones ring and record messages, computers scan data and offer Web pages, and astronomical fees are earned for the parasitical, alchemical art of transforming an object of death into an object of beauty.

"This is where it all happens," Jason tells me triumphantly as we cross into the enforced peace of a cold ice-blue prep room flooded in greenish light. He wears a flamboyant leopard-skin long plastic coat. He is a jumpy, rascally looking boyish man, delighted to show me around. The air is thick, throat-filling. My eyes feel the sting of exposed formaldehyde. The powerful purring AC can't dispose of the malignant odor that calls to my mind every rotting, vile, maggoty thing imaginable. Each breath is like a total immersion in a combustible cruelty. "I like working here," he states simply. "I go home away from the stench anytime I want to. It's an interesting contrast, a healthy way to live." He offers me a Baci chocolate from a box and relates a common prank among interns who perform autopsies: putting a dead severed penis in the lab-coat pocket of a female doctor.

The young female "decedent" on the table has an unexpected embryonic quality: she, or rather, it, both is and isn't human. Whatever makes a human an individual is and is not present in her simultaneously bloated and shrunken, mossy-green body. Dark purple veins marble her chest. Her eyes and ears are thawing. Her skin lifts from her hands and feet, like a snake's discarded sheath. There is nothing sensual or dissolute left in her. She looks terribly sick, Frankensteinian, incomplete—but not alien.

My first thought at the sight of this is that I want to get cremated. My second thought is a feeling: a wave of harrowing awe. And when I've collected myself, I finally know why I am talking to these people: to see what transgression does to the transgressor, to understand the source of our impunity. I've come face-to-face with Babel: the unfathomable constructs of our imagination.

Unlike Courtney, Jason is more interested in the mechanics than in the emotions of preparing the dead. He is not attracted to what he calls the blood and gore. "I see a lot in this job," he chats. "No body is inviolate. A mortician I knew liked to push a trocar [large hollow needle used to suction fluids from corpses] inside every male cadaver's penis and say the stiff had got a boner. I caught him pulling up his pants many times as I came in. I told him off. I'm sentimental about human material. I'm not curious about biology. To me, life is in the appearances. Why do you think we worship Christ on the cross? We identify with the vulnerability. A freshly embalmed body," he sighs, politely covering up the "raw" corpse with a sheet, "is something wonderful. It's like *My Fair Lady:* after I transform death into something lovely and elegant, I feel I own a part of it. And sometimes, if I put a lot of work into it, I hate to part with it. For some minutes, I know unconditional love."

He looks like he never sleeps; his body lacks for sun. I feel something creepy in his intensity, which prevents me from wanting to ever see him again. And he talks constantly and relentlessly, which is draining. "I don't do remains," he boasts, "or obese or autopsied bodies, unless they're prefrozen and formaldehyded, in which case I can work. If guts or melty fat slide out on the floor, I go away. I take pride in what I do. I keep my art pure. I plan my composition, draw it, intuit what will work. Then I put on my Mozart and fall in love. By the end of it, I've humanized them."

It is a fundamental question: Are corpses human or not? There was a time, not long ago, when the existence of the soul was taken for granted, and when surgeons who worked on cadavers were sent to jail. There have been civilizations that could specify with great exactitude when, and if, the spirit ever left its fleshly casing. Like with most things, in our day those definitions have become increasingly blurry. Science has taught us to be pragmatic: it is generally assumed that the instant our hearts stop, we are things again, like the dust we reportedly came from. Our organs travel in Ziploc bags and iceboxes to be planted into the body of another and belong to another; or they are cut out and thrown in a wastebasket, so that a creator like Jason can take what's left and put his vision on it and make it look like a Greek god or a movie star. And then he can fall in love with it, briefly; in love, that is, with his image on the mirror of mortality. Now I know I don't have it in me to watch his ministrations on the defenseless husk of this woman, be they creative or amorous.

When I tell him I must leave, he's gravely disappointed. I have offended and alienated him. I'm surprised he is still vulnerable to the criteria of the outside world, for he has chosen a life of supreme alienation. The very thing that separates us from animals is the consciousness of our mortality, I tell him, which motivates our morality, our ingenuity, and our ability to choose. You may love your job, I say; you may even love these bodies you prettify. But who owns these bodies? Who are they? Are they nothing but other peoples' memories? You're handling human flesh as if it were only meat. Doesn't that give you what we call the fear of God? "I'm not a prude," he says, as if that explains everything. "I understand the utility of death. And I think nothing is unnatural that can be done. I'd say you lack in imagination." I try to imagine a glaring man snorting and huffing, grabbing and pounding into this lifeless flesh, and my mind breaks down mystified. It's the image of utter chaos. And I'm standing too close to it. I can't watch you lay a hand on her, I repeat. "If you're not going to keep a open mind," he says dejectedly, "you won't get any answers. You have to live it, really." What I am facing, I realize, is the culmination of human pathos and prerogative. It is both the epitome and the mutation of our longing to master—I daresay, to "lick"—death. And it could only happen in a time where our freedom is assumed to be absolute, and when nothing seems quite real. And I don't want to live it, really.

Miami and Santa Fe: Alien Romance

> "Nothing exists except atoms and empty space; everything else is opinion."
>
> *Democritus, 362 B.C.*

Reality is the sum of all relationships, and, even in its banality, it is ultimately impenetrable. And perhaps the reason we write books is that the essence of humanity is always fleeting.

The most interesting SAA member I had met while researching sex addiction was a UFO abductee. His promiscuity consisted of having indiscriminate sex with alien abductors; he wanted to quit. I saw his ET fixation as the Kafkaesque revolt of a lonely ordinary individual struggling against obscure powers in an alien world and looking for harmony in the most fantastic places. I didn't think he could find it in support groups because they discouraged the traditional American ideals of diversity, individuality, and chutzpah; they propagated a hermetic, arch, sexless language that was more a mass dirge moan than a relief or a cure. They understood sexuality one desire, and one corresponding rule, at a time.

"When the unifying force disappears from the lives of men and when contradictions lose their context and acquire independence, then the need for philosophy is born," Hegel wrote. The more we keep falsely dividing the world, the more we run after

ourselves, trying to unite our parts as we separate them. But it is in this stray process of chasing and being chased and getting caught between loss and recovery, hunger and disgust, despair and arrogance, between our unquenchable desire for everything and our primal fear of everything, that we transcend our limits. "Once a philosopher, twice a pervert," Voltaire wisely remarked.

I had a prior commitment to go to Miami to meet a conceptual photographer for another project I was considering, so I took the chance to put aside the realities and unrealities of sex in America and just lie on the beach, talk shop, and wait for a private cascading epiphany on how I would bring together this wayward book. On my first day the überhip photographer took me to a pretentious party that was catered by a gay UFO abductee. I like coincidences. They make life interesting and easy. And having a horror of humorless intellectuals, I was innately inclined to abandon the learned photographer for the awed abductee, for whom the UFO world was like the magic phallus of Osiris or Shiva that presented itself as the source of new life.

A Novice's Glossary

RE: realization event (the occasion that triggers an abductee's first memory of having been abducted); regression (the process of recovering repressed memories under hypnosis); memory wipes (the aliens' procedure of erasing one's memory of abduction experiences, which can then only be retrieved in hypnosis); Mindscan (the aliens' ability to read the abductee's mind); stolen/missing time (the abductee's experience of being unable to account for a chunk of recent time); hybrid (half-alien, half-human); OOBE: out-of-body experience.

I've been sleeping with aliens for years," a tall, handsome chef tells me one afternoon in Miami at a Ford models' party. Sampling his culinary wizardry, I had joked that this "roomful of tall, gaunt, dazzling creatures resembles a gathering of aliens—only aliens one would want to sleep with." With carefully tousled hair, bookshelf shoulders, pointy nipples, and cinched waist, his form-fitting Gucci pants and top, Zach blends in. But Zach is serious about sex with extraterrestrials. He tells me hypnosis has "proved" his sexual involvement with alien visitors aboard spacecrafts.

Since 1961, when the Barney and Betty Hill abduction made it into *Look* magazine, thousands of ordinary Americans have provided consistent reports of abduction experiences. MIT physicist Dr. David Pritchard estimates that 1 percent of the nation's population, 2.25 million citizens, are abductees. Other studies place this number between 560,000 and 3.7 million. A 1991 Roper poll revealed that several million Americans may have had abduction experiences. Taking into account that most people never share their stories with analysts, and that most abductions are supposed to be "quick in and outs" (people are collected asleep from their beds and returned with no memory of what transpired), the actual number of sexually used abductees remains incalculable.

The Ford party moves to a cavernous blinking, booming club, Amnesia, where invisible foam machines soak the frenzied crowd in suds and ejaculate-like synthetic rain. I keep sliding on the sodden floor, my clothes clinging to my skin, until Zach suggests we go for midnight lobsters. We cut through a throng of pushy clubgoers, oily dealers and goons, gangly skateboarders, muttering drunks, wide-eyed loiterers in dirt-caked garments and end in a bustling café on Ocean Drive. The street before us is pulsing: Cuban girls in tiny bustiers, sumptuous black men in fashionably untied overalls, strutting gays in dishabille, and ubiquitous coltish models compete for libidinal attention. Here the human body has trumped gravity: mammaries and backsides point uniformly to the sky. The flaunted physicality of this crowd is a modern maenadic celebration of the victory of technology over anatomy.

It's not a far cry from this to shape-shifting beings from other dimensions. Zach, in a mesh top, bangles, and aviator glasses, is telling me about his life. He's thirty-four, the product of a conventional Protestant upbringing. As a child he went to church and believed in the Holy Spirit. He did graduate culinary studies in Hyde Park, married there, and has a nine-year-old daughter. He doesn't consume drugs, alcohol, meat, sugar, caffeine. Some years ago he realized he was gay, but remains close to his wife. "My daughter is the reason I go on living as if none of *this* is happening," he says. "My abductee-mentor, Lee, told me I must make sure my daughter 'knows' and raise her with her alien spirit intact."

Zach's realization event came when he read an article in a local magazine and recognized the abductee symptoms—such as waking up with nosebleeds (ostensibly from nose implants) and tiny unexplained scars or "scoop marks" (from blood-taking or serum-injecting procedures). The reporter referred him to Lee, a local activist who had just attended the 1992 MIT abduction conference sponsored by David Pritchard and Harvard psychiatrist John Mack, which was held on the premise that abductions may be our entry to the science of the twenty-first century. Lee explained to Zach that the magnitude of the abductee phenomenon stays underreported because our anthropocentric pride in being the planet's dominant intelligence, inhabiting a measurable objective reality, is the sacred assumption of our race. Like most credible abductees, Zach had never had exposure to UFO lore. He was apprehensive when he told Lee his recurrent dream of a surreal machine being placed on his penis and his semen being sucked out in a funnel; in response, Lee gave him a copy of Dr. David Jacobs's book, *Accounts of UFO Abductions*.

Dr. Jacobs interviewed abductees from vastly diverse backgrounds, after subjecting them to extensive psychological testing that pronounced them sane. His subjects reported three hundred and fifty abductions that involved interspecies breeding experiments, during which the aliens induced in them rapid, intense, artificial sexual arousal and orgasm, collected their ova or sperm, mixed it with alien DNA, and implanted it back into the women. The impregnated women were reabducted in time to have the hybrid fetus removed. These X-rated spacenappings followed such a familiar pattern that Zach realized his own experience was "like a broken record."

Dr. Jacobs's thesis is that the abductions serve for the production of hybrid children; it is an exegesis Budd Hopkins, an alien-abduction pioneer, introduced in *Intruders*, after studying fifteen hundred cases. Both authors speculate that an alien race has been harvesting our fertility issue in order to replenish its genetic stock after a holocaust that decimated its planet. The abductees feel violated and raped.

Zach disdains this anthropocentric view. He sides with Dr. Mack, who has described aliens as cosmic conservationists and abductees as members of an endangered animal population who are being tagged. The aliens, Zach explains, don't need so many abductees to rebuild their race. Instead, they are preventing our own extinction in an upcoming cataclysm. They're crossbreeding our races until we're indistinguishable, so we can gain their insights. They perform genetic compatibility tests as the first step to an eventual dimensional merging. Hybridization is our species' evolution in progress. Zach now feels pride for his nefarious participation in the salvation of an endangered humanity; since he met Lee and began "contributing willingly," he hasn't had memory wipes.

Ever since he was a toddler, Zach suffered from "old-hag nightmares." "I always saw probing scary eyes, my body prone on an altar or table, and the same terrifying shadowy female raping me, sucking away my essence. Sometimes my testicles were pulled aside and tubes were inserted there. My penis showed signs of having ejaculated when I woke up, but I found no cum. All my life I slept with the lights on, the TV blaring, and tranquilizers." His shrink attributed the dreams to his fear of women and his innate homosexuality. Another therapist suggested Zach might have been sexually handled by his mother as a baby and was suffering from post-traumatic stress disorder. He was prescribed lithium and bipolar-disorder mood stabilizers. Nothing worked.

He lives with a shrink. "We've been monogamous five years, but my lover is increasingly threatened by my alien wife. It's hard to be the spouse of an abductee who's erotically involved with aliens. He's receptive, but it's affecting our sex life, as I spend more and more sexual energy with the entities. He's out cold in bed when I'm ejaculating in space. In the morning, I'm too drained to respond to him. But he knows *they* hold the strings. It's not up to me." He sounds disturbingly sane.

It was only after he met Lee and started undergoing hypnosis that Zach became conscious of his visits with his alien wife—a seven-foot-tall, dark-eyed "guardian angel" with thin silvery-blond hair and a triangular head, who vaguely resembles his ex-wife. ("That's why, when I first saw my ex, I felt I already knew her and loved her.") During regression, he remembers seeing various "Grays" and "Reptilians," but he always mates with the same Nordic humanoid who, he says, originally took his boyhood virginity. "She's my teacher, my sister, my lover, my friend, my soulmate," he gushes, disgorging a loose collection of idyllic clichés. "She's the best part of me. When I look into her huge, oval, nonreflective eyes, I feel she can see all the way through me. Everything goes into slow motion, gets foamy. She's like a daffodil, with no muscles or veins, and yet she is imperious, absolute, and she overpowers me. My stomach gets queasy. My bowels pinch. I feel bliss."

I recognize her as a descendant of the love-goddess born of

sea foam, the siren or mermaid sailors encountered in distant seas. I tell Zach his succubus has been known as Baubo, Brizo, Lilith, Lamia, Brigit, Mirian. Hollywood and a few millennia of mythmaking can easily imprint visions like his on our subconscious. Any contemporary mind, crowded with disparate images of ETs, starving children, *Star Wars*, and Jurassic dinos, could produce these images during sleep or hypnosis.

"But every time I hybridize," Zach insists timidly, "I feel a physical vigor. I don't *imagine* that. I've seen hundreds of fetuses gestating in incubators aboard the craft. I've been shown hybrid toddlers and teens who look human without eyebrows. I was an incubator baby myself, born with no eyebrows; Lee says that shows I'm a dual referencer. My soul is the alien." "Dual reference" denotes the sense of many abductees that they are related to the aliens, much in the tradition of seers taking on the identities of deities or ghosts who speak through them. Some abductees feel they were aliens in past lives. Others, like Zach and Lee, feel they have alien "blood" in them. According to them, our DNA tests are too primitive to register these unconventional genetic nuances.

Zach's fine-featured face contorts when I press him to describe the sex. After a few minutes of unblinking reflection, he grows exhilarated and says: "My body remembers every detail. She is soft. Cold. Yellow. I'm naked. She usually straddles me. My penis feels hollow and flexible, not fully hard. My testicles are little bumps. She fills my mind with spinning erotic images. She's the dominant, even when she props me up on top of her. She stares at me until I know my submission, then rubs against my penis and collects my cum. I don't think they have sex organs, but they create facsimiles for the sex act so we can relate to them. She has breasts. The idea that this superior, refined being is milking my ejaculate is what's terribly arousing. Sometimes when it's time to go, I cry. I feel I'm hers. Nothing in life prepared me for these experiences." That's true of all love, I muse, that doesn't become routine.

"I'm glad you're not gawking in disbelief," he sighs. "I'm sensitive to doubt. I'm still afraid of ridicule. This is a skeptical society, even though you'd die if I told you the names of all the movie stars and police chiefs who are abductees." How come you're not gay in space? I ask. "No one can be. Sex for the sake of pleasure or intimacy alone is foreign to them." His almond eyes keep straying from mine. He looks jittery, haunted. "I know that nothing out there is safe," he adds. "Right before a visitation, I get a dread of apprehension. My heart squeezes shut. It can accelerate into blind panic if I let it."

As I see it, aliens are our ghosts-of-the-moment. Copulating with immaterial species is the postmodern version of being seduced by nymphs, fairies, spirits, and demons. For millennia, people have firmly believed in otherworldly creatures who could kidnap or paralyze innocent or predisposed passersby, stealing their senses and wits or endowing them with supernatural gifts. Until the sixteenth century, madness was a sign of being "touched" by the gods. The UFO is the newest echo of our oldest fear coming down through the bowels of history: We are not safe. By naming our invisible pursuers, we can assuage and define our terrors. By fucking them, we can become them: *we* become miraculous.

Santa Fe looks like a toy town, so uniformly pretty it could be the prototypical Disney-city. My hotel, like every building, even banks and gas stations, is a pink, dainty adobe. The streets are clean and safe, bustling with middle-class tourists, helpful locals, shy Navajos, and well-preserved retirees. Souvenirs include rubber aliens and alien-shaped earrings, cookies, and embryos. I don't find a single properly dilapidated, crude adobe wall to confirm the antiquity of Santa Fe's aesthetic.

Zach's mentor, Lee, and Lee's girlfriend, Jill, are young, New Age retirees. They have turned their back on secular ambitions to do the aliens' bidding: their task is to spawn hundreds of hybrids. "We are the human link," they tell me. "It's our evolutionary mission." They ask me to alter their identities because they are "committed to living outside the corrupting media matrix." "I fear humans more than anything else," Jill gravely explains. They remind me of hardshell missionaries, enthusiasts who would die for their beliefs. Their "metaterrestrials" provide them with a heroic cause that absolves and redeems them from the flat finitude of the quotidian mire. They have left their jobs—he as an electrician and she as a counselor for sexually abused children—and now sell UFO drawings in local galleries, lead "astral therapy" and "hybrid awareness" classes, and "try to live in balance with nature."

Lee picks me up at the Albuquerque airport in a UFO T-shirt, swaggering with open-legged bravado, his camouflage pants tightly sashed at the waist. He has a stubborn jaw, Mongolian eyes, a silver thumb ring, never raises his brittle voice, and spits off-white Skoal gobs into a plastic cup. He sees himself as a spy, "a double agent between worlds." His father was a career military man ("Joe Authoritarian, whipping out his belt if I didn't get an A"). Lee worked as an electrician in his youth, until he was abducted from his truck and returned upside down; later his company sent him to set up lines in Peru, where he had another abduction, during which he was "contracted to an infinitesimal point": "I was returned to bed huddled up in a fetal ball. That taught me to let go of my need for power and control. I refused to lord it over the Incas." Now he drives about chasing hunches, keeping tabs on clandestine government activities against aliens.

His station wagon contains binoculars, tape recorders, CD radios, cameras, UFO magazines, military IDs. His premise is a familiar one, most convincingly presented by Dr. Richard Boylan, a psychologist and outspoken abductee: America's Star Wars defense system is aimed at aliens. That is why, Lee says, SDI funding has increased by 33 percent each year since the Soviet collapse; America has hijacked UFO technology and is building electromagnetic pulse/laser weapons and test-flying noiseless saucers across these desert skies; the government runs a disinformation campaign denying the presence of aliens until it develops weapons to defeat them. In 1994, the government conceded that most UFO sightings of the past fifty years were sightings of secret experimental military aircraft. Still, 49 percent of all Americans believe the government is concealing evidence of alien visitations. John Lear, son of the Learjet founder, has claimed on TV that the government is in possession of the aliens who reportedly crashed at Roswell, New Mexico, in 1947, and they are giving Uncle Sam technology in exchange for abductees. Philip Corso, an Army colonel and author of *The Day After Roswell*, has tried to prove that everything we know about fiber optics, laser beams, and computer circuitry is the result of technology we seized from the crashed spaceship. Roswell's UFO Enigma Museum and International UFO Museum and Research Center are thriving.

The Kirtland air base in Albuquerque houses the Defense Department's Strategic Defense Initiative headquarters, the Sandia National Labs (developing Star Wars weapons), the Defense Nuclear Agency headquarters, and the National Atomic Museum. The National Solar Observatory, the Army Frequency Surveillance Station, and the National Radio Astronomy Observatory are located nearby. The Los Alamos Labs (housing nuclear fusion research centers and the Human Genome Project) and the Tonopah USAF Headquarters and Test Range are within driving distance. This nucleus attracts believers like Lee. He moved here in 1994, after an OOBE abduction in Miami when he was transported to a desert planet he recognized as his alien home. "My planet once had trees and water, but science destroyed it," he says. "We'd made something we couldn't stop. So my new life on earth has to be planetarily useful. I'm a pacifist vigilante."

Recent experiments with electrical disturbances on the temporal lobe of the human brain (the interpretive cortex) have shown that UFO images may be naturally produced effects of high-amplitude electromagnetic pulses caused by tectonic plate movements. People who live near transmitter towers, power lines, fault lines, railway lines, and such, are more vulnerable to them. If radiation is causing a global UFO psychosis, this area is extremely prone. More generally, if any collective disturbance to our subconscious, caused by the impact of modern science on human life, has psychokinetically materialized in an observer-created reality (what Carl Jung called "materialized psychisms"), Lee believes it has come to impart a warning of impending ecological destruction. And if abduction is not a new psychiatric phenomenon or a millennial hysteria, then alien spaceships may be our future intergalactic Noah's ark.

Lee has most of his "encounters" while driving around. This, too, is typical: most people who are not abducted at 3 A.M. from their beds are abducted from their cars on back roads. The person's car (that quintessential American womb-tomb symbol) gets stalled, a crown of dazzling light shines, and a "Gray" being—spineless, hairless, noseless, odorless, genitalless and genderless, four-fingered and big-headed, naked or in a seamless uniform—taps the window or opens the door and, in an indescribable flash of time, an American citizen is transported, floating through a slit, into a luminous cigar-shaped disk and inside the aliens' cold circular labs. The bright flash that persists in the craft resembles near-death experiences and experiences during orgasm. Even the nonsexual encounters qualify as orgasmic, since orgasm is a consciousness-altering experience that can seem "out of body."

These experiences uphold a stalwart religious tradition: Ezekiel in the Old Testament and John in the Apocalypse saw a fiery brightness and winged four-headed humanoids who lifted them up, Emperor Constantine saw a fiery cross in the sky when he conquered Rome, and Joseph Smith saw a pillar of light and two bright creatures in the air who spoke to him. Each of these raptures led to the founding of a church. Like the UFO cultists, early Christians lived in disenfranchised communes and preached of salvation from a corrupt and dying world through abstinence or controlled procreation. Is it a stretch to expect that we may one day be worshiping a boneless Dr. "Gray" and wearing little gold dirigible-shaped disks around our necks, as the ancient Phoenicians and Mythraists once did?

Lee doesn't see abductions as a topical makeover of a timeless anxiety or psychic need. He's even inclined to believe that aliens have been responsible for all the paranormal or divine phenomena in history. I ask: Did aliens appear to Buddha under the banyan tree, Muhammad in his cave, Christ in Egypt, and all the seers who formulated our faiths? Lee enlightens me rigidly: "That is known since the eighties. The origin of all religion may well be E-terrestrial, since they've mastered time. When I describe to you an abduction as sequential/linear, I'm translating it to earthly time. Essentially, their visits these days are a reality check for our planet. They use people like me who are genetically open to them to communicate with us. They're measuring our impulses to determine when it's safe for them to appear to everyone. They come to instruct, like a parent who sees a child going astray."

Christ was also a compassionate consciousness that embodied our physicality in order to bridge, however unsuccessfully, the spiritual and material worlds, and to instruct us how to reconnect with each other at a time of crisis. These latest messengers of a greater intelligence may be the effect of the overwhelming presence of technology in our lives merged with our primal religious instinct. In *The Physics of Angels*, Matthew Fox and Rupert Sheldrake explain ETs as "mechanized" angels. "A spiritual void," Sheldrake writes, "was created when the religious imagination withdrew from the heavens, and science fiction has risen up to fill the gap." When religion was strong and science weak, we took magic for medicine; now we take science for magic. What we "see" depends on the predominant belief structure of our culture. In an age when marvel has been supplanted by machines, when space tourism and human cloning are feasible, when the Genome Project ridicules our spiritual singularity, the UFO represents our restored holy circle. As God has been subsumed by technology, a more powerful technology has to come in to qualify as divine, and defy the inescapable everydayness of our mortal fate.

Lee says I anthropomorphize too much—I try to fit the aliens into what we know. He says I'm just like the Church fathers who condemned Galileo to save their governing laws. So I suggest we talk about the sex instead. "The alien body," Lee replies pedantically, "is subtle—hermaphroditic or neuter. It feels like padded cartilage, pliable. Of course, we have no words for any of this. I could tell you I've fucked protoplasmic cavities and polymer vaginas, I could tell you I've fucked in shuttles, on Mars, floating about, levitating, and it's all as accurate as it's not. They take on host bodies. Our sex union is mystical, like alchemy. Sometimes we lock in embrace and rock. Sometimes we're in the cockpit of a ship orbiting earth, lit by the blues of the control lights, and the alien has gray-blue skin and white pubes and we fuck against the controls and it's so cold I see the steam coming out of my mouth. The most accurate version is when they put a faucetlike device on my dick, connect it to a box with electrodes, and stimulate me into orgasm. Our bodies are not used to such contact—it's sensory-vibrational overload. I feel like the first amphibians who crawled on shore. I come and come." No buttocks, no tits, no food or alcohol, no wrists and elbows and knees and ankles, and he comes? Is this the proverbial mind fuck? "They're conditioning me to survive a nuclear war. The first step is to fuck not with my male eyes but my willpower. When I had sex competitively, it held me captive to the culture. Women took up all my time and turned me into a jealous, paranoid maniac. Now I'm a free man. I can lie next to a naked girl and not be torn by desire or worry about my penis size. I react the same to every corporeal manifestation. I'm on the sexual frontier. And when I come, I have reason. As a donor, I put my seed in evolution." I recognize a familiar doctrine: the first step to eternal salvation is sexual self-control and freedom from the flesh.

Back in Lee's sparsely furnished and TV-less adobe duplex, we find Jill arguing points of abductee scripture with her friend Paula. "I say aliens are drawn to menstruating women, like dogs," Paula is saying. "And I think they know the meaning of rape. Instruments can deform the body. I don't consider that sex. Until I see someone having sex with an alien in plain view, I'll stick to men." Jill is a petite thirty-seven-year-old with a kind, modest face, earnest eyes, and raw, outdoorsy beauty. Paula is fifty-three, moon-faced and pudgy, in starched powder blue slacks and shirt, a high school history teacher.

"It's easier for people on the coasts where the support groups and the Budd Hopkins are," Paula instantly complains to me. "But those are the people who go on the TV shows," Jill interjects. "We face discrimination," Paula persists. "Abductees can't call 911 or an 800 hot line. People sympathize with rape victims, but if you say you were sexually assaulted by aliens, they laugh. All we have is each other." But don't abductees feed on each other's forebodings? Don't other people's stories spark more memories? "My head's being messed with anyway," Paula says. "*They* know everything about me. They stick a thing in my ear and show me pictures. I get panic attacks so bad I need someone to say it's OK. That's the group support. Just touching another abductee is calming."

"I know the Beings mean no harm and that I should feel chosen," Paula continues over nettle tea, after Lee leaves. "But when I'm taken from my ranch up to a lab to have tests conducted on my naked body by aliens, and they insert this gross thick liquid in my mouth and make me swallow, and tie my feet to stirrups and probe my vagina with a tube like I'm a specimen, I feel fear, anger, hatred. I just don't like it. Would you?" I recognize my own fear of dentists and gynecologists: the terror of having cold metal enter prone mortal flesh, orally or vaginally; but despite stories of dentists infecting their patients with AIDS and surgeons amputating the wrong limbs, medicine has programmed us to trust its impersonal practitioners to invade our bodies for our own presumed good. "Aliens do that, too," Jill explains. "The terror stems not from the probes but from the breakdown of our reality if we acknowledge our experiences as real. Our minds can go so far before our self-imposed censorship takes over—because we limit our senses to the credulous. Then we live in pickup anxiety."

"Even after the details of my abductions surfaced during hypnosis," Paula tells me, "I tried to block off the access, never talk about them, not read the literature, ignore it. I told my daughter, who is a nurse, that I was delusional and she should put me on brain pills. I *wanted* to be crazy, to get hospitalized, to get better. Then I caught my three-year-old granddaughter playing with imaginary balls of light 'the gray people' had given her, and talking of white children in a ward up in heaven and of passing through walls. I saw there is no way out. My grandson is on Ritalin. He gets confusional and spaces out. Classic abductee. My father and grandfather used to disappear for hours and not know where they had been. One time Dad came back and didn't need his reading glasses anymore. The last time my grandpa vanished from his car, he never returned. Now my grandkids have relationships with the aliens; I can't spank them and forbid them from talking to strangers, so I have it where I can keep an eye on it. Abduction is generational. My daughter is now writing tons of poems *they*'re dictating to her. She has no choice." I suggest abduction may be a fantastic alternative to routine problematic relationships, a consuming romance at the intersection of science and pop culture; the alien is the abductee's love object and creation in one, an X-rated Tinker Bell–cum-muse; a flawless opiate.

"And how do you explain missing time?" Paula asks. "If you find yourself unable to account for your time, if you're driving continuously and reach your destination two hours later than you should, if you don't recall the last ninety miles, you've probably been abducted, sexually examined, and inseminated." What about sleeping at the wheel, highway fatigue, road mirage, absentmindedness caused by stress or old age? "That doesn't leave you pregnant! After my first lapse, I had nausea, cramps, back pain, swollen breasts, no period. My doctor thought I was with child, but the test kept coming back negative. I had a CAT scan, ultrasound; I thought it was cancer. Under hypnosis, I recalled being on a table and having my fallopian tube artificially inseminated with a painful syringe of sperm." The alien has supplanted the trickster with the lantern who implanted the baby soul, I suggest again.

"In my second trimester," Paula continues excitably, "I was reabducted. They induced labor pains and sucked the halfling baby, while I was bleeding. It was the size of a fist and it had no weight. I didn't want them to do this ever again, so I've had my tubes tied. Since then, they float me up periodically to watch me interact with the baby. I tell it stories, sing to it. I've nursed it." The baby, I muse, is her changeling, her Minotaur; a virgin-birth hybrid that may one day be the messiah of an alien Second Coming. "I'm afraid it's more pedestrian than that," Jill elucidates. "We all have our jobs up there. Because with knowledge comes responsibility. Paula is a Caregiver. Lee is a Teacher: he educates new abductees on nonlinear time structure and ego-surrender. I'm an Empath; they are training me to replace people's fear with trust telepathically. Our basic lesson is unconditional, unlimited, eternal love. The second lesson is to be prepared—for the breakdown of all life."

• • •

When she was six, Jill went camping with her father; one night she felt him come into her sleeping bag and sexually penetrate her. She didn't speak on the way home and, some years later, after undergoing incest memory retrieval, she stopped speaking to him altogether. Her family, a clan of philanthropists from the Rockies, resented her accusations and saw her as a black sheep. When she was thirty, she immaculately conceived. *Her* test came back positive. She had an aversion to being sexually touched all her life and hadn't been sexual since she "reclaimed the incest wounds." Baffled, she read on blighted ova and pseudocyesis, and chanced upon Jacobs's reports on "the missing fetus syndrome," a physical aftereffect of abductions. She recalled that, before her pregnancy, she had had erotic dreams that involved penetration. Three months later, she was not pregnant. Her doctor thought it had been ectopic, but she had no miscarriage, bleeding, or discharge. She decided it was a question of interpretation. She underwent hypnosis. "I recalled the Beings telling me about universal motherhood," she says. "We conversed telepathically. ESP is the purest form of communication; there's no room for lies. They apologized for putting me in my dysfunctional family: they explained they had orchestrated my conception for a worthy reason. I felt held in the light."

Some psychiatrists believe that ET sexual memories, like ritual abuse memories, are common outcomes of childhood abuse. Abused children dissociate from their grim physical realities by creating an alternative fantasy world to inhabit, where they can feel special. As adults, they blame their uneasiness and anxiety about sex on alien or ritual abuse. Jill feels her case disproves this: under hypnosis, she remembered her first alien "insemination" had happened on her camping trip with her father. "I was little and the needle hurt me badly, so I had blamed my earth dad for not protecting me. I was relieved to learn I wasn't molested by him. I felt grateful to them for opening my eyes. The pain was necessary to penetrate the density of my denial. It helped me undergo tremendous personal growth. I felt compelled to dedicate my life to helping others come to terms with this."

Until then, she had been terrified of sexual intimacy. During sex, she used to lie paralyzed, feeling used and powerless; she felt safe only when she said no to a man. "I realized sex brought back the fears I had when I was first abducted. That healed me. Now an alien can touch me on the forehead with its longest finger and I orgasm." Jill claims to have incubated forty-two hybrids. Sometimes she is taken to a maternity ward and picks out her offspring by smell. She has mated with dazed male abductees ("We don't speak; he enters me, does his thing, and walks off") and hybrids ("Sexual dysfunction is a problem of hybrids, so the doctors check if a hybrid can reach ejaculation, and retrieve it from me to test the sperm count"). It seems to me aliens behave as badly as the worst deadbeat human males: abduct, hurry the act, dump. I ask about her sex life with Lee. She looks at me as if I come from another planet. "We have soulmate sex. We've learned it from the aliens. The [alien] penis is a light fluctuating contour of energy. It's nothing like coarse human sex. Nothing personal is at stake." Europa was raped by a bull and spawned a continent, Semele was raped by golden rain and gave birth to Bacchus; our interspecies sexual abductions weren't always so numinous or hygienic. It seems even our most symbolic forms of self-expression are vulnerable to the wave of public moral-health censorship that has surged throughout America.

Jill suggests we spend the night at the mesa where she had her most recent encounter. We pack sleeping bags and drive through a majestically stark, desolate landscape. She says she and Lee see them every day. Some come from hundreds of millions of miles away. Some are busy, effective technicians; others are loving, benevolent allies. She sees them so easily she can channel them at will. "It's reassuring to be with them; but if I have to focus on my consensus reality, I screen them out. If you really look, you'll see one behind that bush over there watching us." I only see tangled nightfall-gray shadows.

"Do you feel you belong to this world?" she asks. I have moments when I don't recognize my surroundings, I admit. "Did you feel watched as a child?" I was impressionable, I say; I "saw" baleful Boschian creatures hiding in shadows and sometimes made up stories about them. In this voguing world, we know we count if we are watched. "My intuition knows a contactee," Jill exclaims. "You'll know what it is when they come, *if* they haven't come already. Try hypnosis." But do you feel *desire* for them? I ask, deflecting the issue. "If I don't have an interaction, I feel undernourished, neglected, unloved. I yearn for them. Lee loves me, but this is a bigger cosmic love. When I'm with them, I feel larger than I am, electric. My body bursts into a million pieces of light, free of the physics that limit us. The human body is such a poor piece of machinery compared to the soul. So I give them my body, and they give me their wisdom. We're all extraterrestrial in a way: our psyches are not confined to earth."

I don't believe it's our bodies that fail us. I think of how the charisma of a repressed homosexual renamed Do, the passage of the Hale-Bopp comet, and the existential anomie of living "in no context" led the Heaven's Gate cult in San Diego to deliver themselves of their problematic earthly "vehicles" by committing mass suicide in 1997. Their Web site was marked with a doe-eyed glowing alien. Their message was obedience, brotherhood, and castration. I think of the Raelian cult, whose 35,000 members believe that cloning is the key to eternity, the Bible was written by aliens, every miracle can be attributed to technology, and that our age of Revelation, entered in 1945 with the bombing of Hiroshima and man's mastery of matter, will culminate in the coming of our alien creators by the year 2035 when we're technologically ready. I wonder why even people who view the soul as DNA espouse the abductees' vision of a hybridized "single-multiversal" future that echoes the Christian promise of heaven. I can only reason that, as the unconfirmable joys of heaven convinced hundreds of generations to do without the joys of life, so our aliens reinforce our superstitious puritanism that puts duty above pleasure and mind over body and sex back in the brig of procreation.

In his book *The Religion of Technology*, historian David Noble has proposed that Western religion and technology have been feeding off one another for a millennium, with the result that modern technology "remains suffused with religious belief." By religion, he refers to Christianity, with its perfectionist work ethic and its belief in an eventual restoration to the original unsullied life of Eden. According to Noble, from the Middle Ages onward, technology became eschatology. The Church sanctioned man's domination of the natural world and draped technology with an apocalyptic destiny that came down to us as the authoritative mythology of progress. Noble warns that, instead of serving our needs, "the technological pursuit of salvation has become a threat to our survival."

We're still helpless before the physical world. We can't control our bodies. Haunted by our desire for unalloyed mastery, worried about the future of our children, we look for new archetypes; and we find them in ultra-advanced intelligences that ironically confirm that we are not in control. We construct myths of abduction and powerlessness because we sense that we can never catch up with our technologized new world that's ruled by lab-dwelling scientists we don't understand.

So Jill and I recline under an expanse of shimmering billion-times-billion stars and whisper like girls at a slumber party. I tell her science says everything alive traces its ancestry to a bacterial cell that combusted 3.5 billion years ago, whose genetic code we all share; our bond with the planet is in our bodies. What we really are is flesh that can dream. She tells me stories of flying with her aliens in the moonlight over dunes and clinging to them to keep from falling, and my eyes widen. Starry nights evoke our inconsequence, our living in the proverbial colony of fleas on an elephant's hide—thinking everything has been ordained for our existence, until the elephant sneezes. I see a dozen mutely falling stars.

The two of us lie in wait, hunters of an ingenious exotic prey, pretending to be falling asleep. Hours pass. I'm not roused by any white light. Suddenly Jill, I think in desperation, knowing I'm leaving the next day and wanting me to bear witness, goes into a trance. Her eyelids flutter, her eyes glimmer half-shut, her body shakes vehemently, insensible to my comforting touch. Her lips move with the economy of a ventriloquist's, as her firm counselor's voice shifts into the voice of a little girl (who I understand is Jill), an old man (a doctor-mentor who sounds as if he's coming through a scrambler), and a general "we," ethereal and playful (who must be the hybrids). The voices communicate vague directions for my future ("trust in the universe; follow your heart") accented with fairly accurate details from my past and also from past lives I can't verify. Jill sobs, pants, and empathizes, then sighs and smiles benignly, looking utterly cleansed and blissful. When she comes to, she says that my eyes sparkle "reensouled," lucid and bright like the stars. I sleep like a baby, free of dreams.

Memphis: Hypercoitus

"The imagination is the spur of delights; everything depends upon it, it's the mainspring of everything."

Marquis de Sade, Philosophy in the Bedroom

We're a cockteased culture, predicated on the triadic tyranny of profit, comfort, and illusion, versed in the use of antiseptic condoms and technofetishisms, lusting after aliens or screenal bodies of media stars, sampling simulated sex in strip joints, video orgies, or tiny MUDs. In fact, cybersex is the best example of our vicariousness: it is both a conduit of sexual freedom (freedom from identity, bodily constraints, repercussions, stereotypes, guilt) and an outcome of our lack of freedom (simulation is safer than reality, and only metaphor is truly "safe sex"). The Net allows the body to love itself by letting it be rid of itself: plugged into circuit boards, it's finally free to find ecstasy. By prizing the imagination over the senses, and transporting pleasure beyond the realm of the flesh, hypersex is the most representative sex of our time, at once unrepressed and puritanical. It's the fairyland of Neither/Nor.

Ever since my trip to Provincetown, I had sustained a cyber-affair I didn't quite know was one. When I returned from Europe, it reached a crescendo and, to my surprise, had to be resolved. It would have stayed a private affair if I had been able to consummate it, but the only thing I could do with words was write. After all the time I had spent on this project, it felt natural when I met my cyberlover that I should interview him. I was used to being an observer; my writing on sex had kept me out of the mating game, for writing always isolates us and even chains us where we hope to be set free. And this is the very paradox that defines life on the Internet.

Since I can remember, I've read everything that comes my way. I read junk mail, flyers I'm handed in the street, toothpaste tubes and soap boxes, every novel and magazine I can, encyclopedias, congressional records, dictionaries, annotated papers, many of them many times, and each time I don't put them down until I'm finished and they're always real to me. I read to ground myself and remember the world I am part of, and I read to forget the immediate small sense of life, and, as I am always reading, my friends quip I must join Readers Anonymous to cure my inertia and acquire a short attention span. But I couldn't read the chat-room texts, even after I printed them out. They were missing something elemental that I couldn't do without: authorial intent. I realized that the dehumanization of expression that characterizes our century, initiated by creative writers who felt alienated, was now adopted by millions of individuals as their uniform expression of first-person freedom. The Net seemed to me the site of a society in the process of fleeing itself.

And I couldn't treat those endless cybertexts as spontaneous conversations. When we resort to words, we touch each other only metaphorically: to produce a single, precise word we must stay apart, critical. I'm used to talking with many people and being interested in everything they say and all the while being alone with language; this proclivity should have served me well in cyberbia, but it didn't. Because what interests me most in face-to-face interaction are the gaps and mines between words—the speaker's nonverbal tensions and limitations that complement or reverse the spoken meaning.

I often envy crusaders who find redemption from meaning-
lessness in gifting their energies to animal rights, environmen-
tal protection, starving children, gay liberation—the list is
always long. But I feel I can't do my writing justice if I take up
another cause. And having been a student and a teacher most of
my life, I don't believe anybody teaches anyone anything by
design. Yet I felt so strongly about the absence of the body in
cybersex, about the essential contempt for the body latent in the
sexualities I saw all year, and about our orgiastic merging of
totalitarianism and nihilism that passes for emancipation, that
I found myself imprisoned by a perception that would settle for
nothing short of a revolution in the sexual consciousness of our
time, with an ardor resembling a cause. "Because things are as
they are, they will not stay as they are," wrote Bertolt Brecht.

A Novice's Glossary

MUD, or Multi-User Dungeon (a simulated on-line envi-
ronment, such as a medieval castle or a Hugh Hefnerish
bed, where people can engage in role-playing games or
real-time unsupervised private chat); virtual (the simu-
lated reality that computer connections create); Net (the
Internet, originally a communications system developed
by the Defense Department to use in the event of a
nuclear war); cyberspace (the term, coined by science fic-
tion author William Gibson in his novel Neuromancer,
refers to the collective on-line universe); c-sex, or cybersex
(simulated sex through typed text transmitted over com-
puter networks; also e-sex, for electronic sex, and Net-
sex); Usenet (an Internet forum of many discussion
groups known as newsgroups); BBS, or Bulletin Board
System (an alternative to national servers; the user dials
into the computer to get information or services); chat
mode (a feature of a BBS or national server that allows
one-on-one [or more] live real-time conferencing; also

known as chat rooms, e-rooms, e-chat, c-chat, and hot
chat if the discussions are of erotic nature); F2F (face-to-
face); s2s (skin to skin); r/l (real life); v/t (virtual time).
Some common acronyms of Netspeak: IRL (in real life);
LAFS (love at first sight); RP (romantic partner); SO
(significant other); TL&EH (true love and eternal happi-
ness); LO (lust object); DMV (dreaded monogamy virus);
SMV (sexual market value); NIFOC (nude in front of the
computer); WTF (what, or who, the fuck); LOL (laugh-
ing out loud); <g> (grin). Example of an emoticon: :-)
(smiley face).

"Meet me or kill me, Scheherazade," the message read. I flew to Memphis.

Memphis in spring is blooming with pastel azaleas, hydrangeas, poplars, magnolias, dogwood, drooping willows. It is an orderly, sleepy metropolis with a run-down fragility—moldy arched balconies, brick mansions in over-grown lots, and millionaires with bulky antediluvian cars—a creaky, unironic city, populated by people who prefer spiritual revivals to surgical face-lifts and feel at peace with lassitude and anonymity and appreciate temporal reticence and eti-quette.

I'm here to meet Virgil, who is eager to consummate our "c-affair." He shows up in a Ralph Lauren chalk pinstriped suit and shined Bruno Maglis, and avoids my gaze as he hands me a computer-printed itinerary that includes a visit to Grace-land and annotates my free time with "V. in meeting," "V. with his kids." As president of an alumni association, V. is used to handling visitors who may contribute to the million-dollar endowment. He's surprisingly handsome given the homely stereotype of cyberlovers, with a well-lined face, a lustful mouth, moist eyes, a tall physique, and the manner of an autocrat, curt and disenchanted. When I propose to interview him, he turns defensive, and feeble hints of a southern accent creep into his diction. Then he offers to massage my headache away.

Our cyberaffair began by accident, as most affairs do. I was looking for a school friend and e-mailed Virgil, who turned out to be a stranger of the same name. I apologized and he wrote back commenting on a T. S. Eliot quote in my message. He included a quote by Baudelaire ("If the dull canvas of our wretched life / is unencumbered with such pretty ware / as knives or poison, pyromania, rape / it is because our soul's too weak to dare!"). After that we irregularly exchanged poetic quotes—mine variable and spawned by linguistic pleasure, his consistently erotic. Literature protected us from the forced smart-assed witticisms typical of e-mail exchanges. Still, he was courting me. By the time I realized it and told him I was a cybervirgin, he unfussedly confessed he was in "love."

He didn't know my appearance, my marital status, or my history and didn't ask; he didn't try to meet or shock or impress me. He wanted hyperconsummation. He gave me sensual e-massages (". . . oil flowing down your shoulders, pooling in the small of your back, your hair falling forward, revealing the curve of your nape, earning a sigh from your throat"), and exalted our "Net chemistry" ("I can feel your body language, the very taste of your vibe"). He never mentioned his "r/l."

I realized the Net is giving fresh meaning and validity to the wintry cliché of blind love because the medium encourages a fictional configuration of love and allows romance to remain ideal, untarnished by the abrasions of reality and gravity, hypothetically "true." The resurgence of romantic love generated by this faceless contact and the tales of people leaving spouses for whoever typed the right words on their screens confirm that our greatest love is our love of illusion. What really turns us on is what we imagine.

Virgil had struck me as an appropriate guide into the cybersex underworld, if only by virtue of his eloquence. I followed his lead, being determined to have Net-sex in order to understand it; but I did wonder why he chose to painstakingly seduce and assure me specifically, when millions of ready sexual partners crawled the Net. I could only assume he was a committed cyber-Casanova who enjoyed the obstacles of (textual) conquering more than the quick gratification of a chat-fuck.

But the affair floundered. He is a planner. I don't premeditate. I am a two-finger typist. He types eighty words a minute. When I travel, I don't check my e-mail. He does twice a day. I don't save it. He practically memorizes his. And there were greater discrepancies. No matter what transgressive erotic scenario he typed, it aroused my curiosity but not my senses. I didn't get wet by reading, "I'm licking your lips," or when typing, "I'm licking your balls." I know sex to be impulsive, muddied up, prelingual, and even ferocious, driven by visual and pheromonal cues, centered on the reactions of infinitesimal nerves and blood vessels throbbing beneath skin. For me, sex is a blackout of meaning. "Describe your balls," I typed, in valiant effort. My fingers tapped keys. Dots connected to dots, 1's and 0's poured out into the void. "Hot and heavy," he replied, "nearly bursting." It evoked nothing sentient.

I don't object to sex as anonymous physical therapy. I didn't mind that Virgil didn't know me and had never seen me, that I didn't know him. Desire can be heedless. I minded the lack of substance. I was the immaterial object of an immaterial man's desire. I had no skin, no hair, no gaze, no bone structure. My body wanted to crash through the monitor and put an end to all the words. But I worried that, by assuming sex has to be physical, I neglected that individuals differ in sexual needs as much as in physiognomies. The world was changing so fast that I knew many of my ideas could be out of date before I fully formulated them. For the first time I had to ask myself: Am I conservative? Repressed?

But even if my fingers were fitted with sensor gloves and my head with goggles that could transmit my sexual desires, their message would be untranslatable. Language is a polite compromise, a social tool used for collaboration or persuasion or as a means of comforting our daily panic. But the most poetic or automatic prose is impersonal and endlessly limiting compared with the indescribable discourse of our anatomies. Virtual sex is fiction whereas actual sex is the irruption of the unrepresentable. Because I like sex to stay beyond rational definition, and because I wasn't going to fake an orgasm on the Net, I admitted to my correspondent my electronic frigidity. In cybercockteased desperation, like a lover brought to the point of orgasm and denied, Virgil begged me to fly out.

It is only in Memphis, interviewing him under a pseudonym after he checks on my credentials, that I learn he is a pillar of his community, attends Sunday Mass, hobnobs with heads of foundations and philanthropists, has married into a venerable family, raised beautiful children, and made his parents proud. He is a Boy Scout, a Big Brother, a Phi Beta Kappa, a literacy volunteer, a museum patron, a hospital trustee—and he's lonely. Although he and his southern-belle wife have not been sexual for years, he does not feel safe having an affair, so the Net has been his hormonal outlet. And he's had enough cyber-one-night-stands to quench his lust. "I'd been married so long," he recalls, "I was afraid I didn't know how to date; but I saw all I had to do was write what I wanted to do. It was unbelievable. I became a stud, making love to whoever would respond. Different women, sizes, ages, occupations, saying things they would never have said had we met in person. I didn't have to worry about my smell or clothes or how to hold her hand or being misunderstood. No cat-and-mouse games. They were hot, and honest about it, and wanted to feel desired and desirable, as I did. Their excitement was usually enough to arouse me. And there was always someone new.

"Then I saw how meaningless and demeaning it was," he goes on. "These were idiots who couldn't even spell, first of all, and second they might be lonely homosexuals posing as liberated bombshells, and I ate their menstrual blood or fistfucked them. It disgusted me; I hated all the verbal rape, and I never stopped being afraid of exposure and disgrace even though I used an alias and P.O. address. I quit; but I kept fantasizing about Net-sex when I masturbated, because it was all I had had for so long. I dreamed of a Net-partner I could trust and respect. It seemed impossible until your e-mail. I knew you were who you claimed to be because you were reaching out to an old friend. I had your age, gender, interests, wit, in two lines. Maybe I was conceited, but I instantly conceived a furtive affection for you. If I could cybermarry you, I would be a happy man." I ask what he fell in love with. My name? My drove of quotes? "I found the accident of our connection reassuring," he replies, "*willed* by the Eros of cyberheaven. When words are all you have, you can go deep very fast. The other has got you by the brains." But I'd sent him lines written by dead men. "You chose what you sent me. Your soul was in those quotes." And what if I were repulsive? "That's the point of the Net. We see what we look like mentally, without the constraints of a society that judges people by appearances. It's a communication free of the trappings of the body. I didn't expect to meet you, so your physical being was irrelevant." I tell him I think his quixotic love, of which he is so vain, has nothing to do with me, except that it puts me in the terrible position of being unreasonably loved.

He sighs defeatedly and sits on my hotel bed. A Southern Baptist prone to guilt, Virgil feels his sexuality as a vulnerability, a dereliction of his civic duty; but at the same time his good deeds and forceful words leave him sensually starved. This contradiction makes him a typical cybersex user: his manhood is duty-bound, his flesh neglected, his lust adolescent. A trademark of Net-chat is a sophomoric interest in sex and double entendre, which normally seems more suitable to sexually curious youths keen to express conflicting longings than to social echelons. Another trademark is cybertrust: the leap of faith wary adults won't make in real life but will under-take in a world of unreliable narrators, trusting the written word more than the evidence of their senses. When their phys-ical self isn't the source of attraction, people ironically shed a lifetime's suspicions, heedlessly believing what they can't smell, touch, or see—spurred perhaps by some ingrained faith in word-driven advertising.

This was how Sharon Lopatka and Robert Glass, over-weight, middle-aged strangers, fell in cyberlove—he as "Slow-hand" typing from a trailer in Lenoir, North Carolina, she as "Nancy" from Hampstead, New Hampshire. In 1996, Sharon took a train to Lenoir. When her body was dug out of his yard, Glass, a county-government computer programmer, claimed she died by accident while they were having sex. Their e-mail had touched on torture, bondage, and death. A letter she left behind read: "If my body is never retrieved, know that I am at peace." Possibly, what killed her was her romantic trust in words out of context, her firm reliance on mutable fantasy.

I can tell Virgil wants to touch me, but he's so in control of himself that he feels self-conscious and breaks into a harsh laugh instead. He wants to be capable of a radiant, penetrating love. But he has stepped out of his generally harmless world into circumstances that are unimaginable: the density of my presence throws him off. He seems to fear he may betray him-self and tell me everything he's never said to anyone or be unable to speak because everything true is unsayable. He strategically repeats the small ringing words he's only written before: "I love you." There is both an imperative and a bleat-ing tone in his strong sentimental appeal to me to step into his foggy dream of our bond, but the senselessness of those words startles me, shattering the very mood he wants to establish—the sense of magic at work.

Later that day we bask in the sunshine around Elvis's little fountain, headphones on, listening to an obligatory tape recit-ing the King's riches, when, apropos of nothing, Virgil swings me off my feet and bestows an amiably deranged face on mine, forcing his tongue through my lips in full view of the other tourists, who look away. His face is still burrowed into mine when I repeat my bookwide rule: I can't get involved with my literary subjects. He lifts me onto his shoulder and strides off toward the Graceland bus. "But I'm a *virtual* subject," he protests in a hoarse whisper, and in this simple angry statement resound all the confusion, indulgence, and easy rationalization that are the Pandoran gifts of the Net.

I first heard about cybersex from an avant-garde videomaker back in the Stone Age of the Net. He'd just returned from his first consummating trip, having borrowed his parents' old Chevy and driven across five states to meet a woman who had typed "Come, now." He reportedly left the motor running until they climaxed on her living room floor. "We didn't say hi. The car door stayed open while we grabbed each other and ran to the couch," he gloats three years later. Ira is a fast-talking, unkempt, teddy-bearish media artist in his fifties with a penchant for spilling his guts. "By the end, we were tying each other up. We did everything we'd written about, even pissplay. The sex was great, but she was hysteric. She didn't want me to have sex with other women; she left her husband for me. That was a real tragedy, and I learned my lesson. I'd love extreme sex in real life, but it comes with complications. Now, as soon as it gets real, I stop the connection. The edge is no longer there anyway. In the end, every one of us is pathetic beneath the mask." I guess that the mask is what counts.

Ira really learned his lesson after half a dozen similar encounters. "I drove to Kentucky, Carolina, Delaware, Toronto, Nova Scotia, always worried I'd disappoint them, always disoriented by the real presence of someone I'd been so intense with. I felt like a sex doctor, flying in to fix them up. The Delaware one was a thirty-one-year-old virgin, a disastrous past, naive, and jumpy. The Kentucky one was a librarian, forty-four, living with her kids, very attractive but sexually dull. The Toronto one was gay; I was her first male. But sex is about projection. In the end, face-to-face contact permanently contaminates the relationship on the screen or phone—it becomes unmysterious. All the cybermates I've had eventually wanted a commitment, even if they had manufactured identities. So now I give no information about myself. If I'm pressed, I give a grand tale of intrigue. It's the ability to cut off communication that keeps cybersex positive for me. Inaccessibility is intoxicating. Words alone get the women ready. It's enough to tell a story about someone watching us or tell them to shove their hand up their ass, to get them to come on their keyboards." So the Net is the latest incarnation of the dildo: a talking, two-way sex aid. "It's ideal communication: with one hand you create, with the other masturbate," Ira confirms. "I believe in what the Hungarian psychiatrist Thomas Szasz said: 'Masturbation is the primary sexual activity of mankind. In the nineteenth century, it was a disease; in the twentieth, it is a cure.' America is about freedom."

Hot chat was launched in 1979, when the Source offered an on-line "parti" line that elicited such an immediate consumer response that Net-sex loomed as America's latest land of opportunity. CompuServe, which started in 1969 as a time-sharing service for mainframe computer wireheads, bought the Source in the eighties and popularized its CB Simulator chat playpen. Soon Prodigy, Quantum, Delphi, GEnie, and other on-line ventures offered "health spas," "hot tubs," and private e-rooms. In 1993, America Online was launched; by 1996, it had 7 million subscribers and revenues in excess of $1 billion—most of it from sex-chat, which nets AOL a low estimate of $7 million a month. *Love at AOL*, begun in February 1996, is the service's most heavily used content area, receiving 700,000 visits a month. On a typical Saturday night, 8,000 public, member-only, or private AOL chat rooms are open at once. Ten to 15 million of the 35 to 40 million people cruising the Net every day are chatters, and the number of new sub-scribers is still growing at about 2,300 percent a year. A 1995 Carnegie Mellon report calculated that 83.5 percent of all Usenet images (circulating mostly in Usenet's twenty thousand chat groups) are pornographic, and that trading in sexually explicit imagery is "one of the largest (if not the largest) recreational applications of computer networks." In 1998, a run-of-the-mill request for X-rated images can get fifty thousand calls a month and 2 million log-ons, and an average searcher can download three hundred files of binary nude pictures in an hour. The sexual traffic throughout the Net is unthinkably massive and restless.

Overnight, cyberliving has become chic: the hottest new club in New York is Mother, which caters to Click+Drag—a "safe, family-like, cyberfetish" scene made up of "gender-hackers," "glam nerds," omnipierced punks, trannies, and computer engineers. Its setting is faux-cyber, its clientele wear six-inch chromecone breasts with rubber hoses coiling from them and self-parodying nerdy glasses, the music is industrial house, big screens flash subliminal messages, and a massive TV plays a live feed from a bird's-eye camera that records everyone present, which inspires the clientele to vogue and pantomime. It's a real-world simulation of virtual interactivity.

The culture's cybermania is everywhere: "Boyfriend Tam-agotchi" is the hot new grown-up craze made for Nintendo's handheld Game Boy, whose Operation Boyfriend Makeover involves molding one's digital suitor into the perfect mate with advice, stimulating talk, gifts. Major publishers market Internet erotica books like Mary Anne Mohanraj's Web site stories, titled *Torn Shapes of Desire*, or *Exegesis*, a love story by Astro Teller written in e-mail messages; *Looking for Love Online*, by Richard Rogers, dispenses advice on safe Net-love and on how to "sniff out phonies"; *Love Online*, by Sally Banks, tells the story of how the author found the love of her life on the Net. Madison Avenue is investing in wearable biosensors, and

MIT's trendsetting Media Lab has been staging fashion shows of "translator jackets," Levi's jeans–cum–musical synthesizers, eyeglass monitors, shoetap databases, and costumes that count calories and change color according to one's mood. The hipper students on the hipper campuses already wear their computers strapped to their belts so they can be connected to the Net every waking hour, and tap on one-hand keypads called Twiddlers so they can write their papers while strolling through the park; they call themselves cyborgs—part human, part machine—and espouse Isaac Asimov's view of the future: "If we're lucky, the computers will keep us on as pets."

Gordon is a mudder like Ira, a short, pudgy, shiny-faced twenty-nine-year-old recording engineer who spends up to six hours a day at his computer as a woman. Mudders prefer MUD/MOOS and Talker-MUSHs for "TinySex" because they mistrust giant servicers. "In ten years, America will be an Internet-police state," Gordon says. "The Net is all about manipulation; it's a reclassification of information and power." For now, he trusts himself to outsmart any new system.

"I run up huge bills," Gordon admits, "but if I cut down, I'd be suicidal." He's an extraordinarily low-key, gentle little man. "It's like any social gathering," he says earnestly, "except you can control your image. I run into people from all walks of life here—most are twenty to forty, affluent, educated, overworked, solid professionals for whom dating isn't easy. People who have spent a lifetime looking for the right mate find a compatible SO on-line because here they can communicate undistracted for hundreds of hours without disapproving moral codes, or shame, or body-image crap. This is mainstream America. The world of e-sex *is* the real world, only it's everywhere at once." To me, it sounds icily abstract.

Because the great majority of sex players are male, many men masquerade as female to stand out or for the sport of deceiving other men or out of curiosity about gender-bending.

Some find it relaxing, enlightening, even life-changing. It is reportedly common practice among prisoners. The hoax is so widespread that seasoned players assume heavily flirtatious females are real-life males. Experts estimate that two out of three "women" in sex-oriented chat rooms are men. MIT psychology professor Sherry Turkle, author of *Life on the Screen*, likens Net encounters to psychoanalysis, in which patients project their desires onto remote analysts; Net-deception, Turkle argues, is self-projection (Freud's reality principle).

"Impersonating is a high," Gordon explains. "Female-presenting players are called to 'prove' their gender; if you get found, you're shunned. It's a dare I couldn't win in three dimensions. I've posed as a black dom, had lesbian three-somes, dyke amputee sex. It's reawakened my sex life. Usually I'm a blond vixen with supermodel legs and dazzling green eyes named Alice, after the Wonderland. I model her on the TV character Xena. Sometimes I'm a horny Chicana. When I'm an Asian thirteen-year-old, I get the most graphic mail. I've built these multiple selves and grown used to living with them like characters in an erotic epistolary novel I write. I use garters and stockings to masturbate in, for verisimilitude. I have fantastic orgasms. Anonymity freed me from my inhibitions. It's been so empowering. The Net is a great space for the body." Isn't he confusing the body with a murky idea glowing on a screen? Isn't Net-sex a verbal substitute for sex, a nullifying compromise between our sexual and social desires? "If the woman who understands you better than anyone ever has is a forty-nine-year-old, three-hundred-fifty-pound bald man, what's the difference?" he retorts. "So you're married for twenty-five years, discover chat, and fuck men on-line; it doesn't mean you're gay. It's the arrival of a transgendered world, where we define ourselves not by our physical bodies but by the on-line representations we choose. Multiple personalities will soon no longer be a symptom of madness but a conventional way of living. It's new, uncharted territory."

Apparently, the biggest attraction of cybersex is the freedom to say and be anything one is not—implying that we don't much like what we say and are. Net-sex is mainly a fanciful form of self-love. Most people don't lust after the person they correspond with, but after the persona they create for themselves—their redeeming riposte, self-hype, and wish-projection, which e-pen-pals make sufficiently real. By encouraging us to reinvent ourselves, the Net offers us the traditional American dream—the measureless freedom to be anyone, dazzling and changeable like a movie star. Ironically, this makes the Net an instrument for the dissolution of identity and the proliferation of loneliness: in essence, we're all free to hallucinate the world and disappear in our conjurations of each other.

Adam is a victim of cybersexual transvestism. He is the ambitious thirty-nine-year-old manager of a trade press, telegraphic and fidgety, in chinos, Rockports, a Supercut buzzcut, and a ubiquitous cellular against his ear. In cybertopia he favors Humphrey Bogart suits, raincoat, and hat, and works as an indomitable detective in a virtual town that has its own laws and police system. As its resident P.I., Adam has the opportunity to be exonerated of his real life.

Adam had all his sex on company time ("C-sex is the only sex still possible in the workplace"), until he got seduced by an electronic heavy-breather who proved to be his ideal girl. "She was there every day, attentive, supportive, appreciative. She was only a postal worker, but so voluptuous and sweet, I did something that months earlier would have been unimaginable: I offered to meet her in a hotel room. I was shy. I brought flowers." She turned out to be a burly man in Santa Claus drag who clasped handcuffs on Adam, tied him to the bed, and forced him into a bloody "erotic exploration of rape." The story of Oliver Jovanovic, the Columbia doctoral student charged with kidnapping and sexually assaulting a Barnard student with whom he had an on-line affair, was in the news. But Adam was too ashamed of his abuse to turn to the law, and he didn't know the identity of his molester. "I still often run into some-one on-line I know is evil, a Dahmer-type geek who makes my skin crawl," he adds. Adam's company requires its personnel to take an Internet-sensitivity course, and supervisors can spy employee e-mail for signs of sexual harassment.

Adam's sex life now revolves around a $5-a-minute ($50 for thirty minutes) service that provides female models who per-form live private striptease on his screen. He tells them what to take off, what body parts to have the camera zoom in on. "It's a cheap and convenient date," he says, considering the strip-pers will congenially hear his most profound thoughts while they perform requested gyrations. The video technology is primitive, an eery spasmodic display of ten stills a minute, but he assures me "it's addictive."

Joel is Adam's colleague, an editor who just received his master's from a virtual college. He's thirty-six, happy-looking and roly-poly, with a reassuring purry voice, wavy silver hair, and a shocked expression. He has developed severe carpal tunnel syndrome from Net-sex, and blithely describes the excruciating wrist pains, the expense of posture courses and safe equipment, the sex-withdrawal symptoms. Before his afflic-tion, he had 19 cyberaffairs and 231 cyber-one-night-stands. He kept a detailed log of his lovers' predilections, like a serious col-lector. He never saw them off-line after an early hurtful deser-tion: the one woman he had met excused herself to get her nude shots from her car, and never came back. He knew why: he wasn't what she had expected from his e-persona.

I ask how he became a winning hyper–Don Juan. "I wrote out a list of all the things I didn't have the nerve to do in person. I wrote down the qualities I found lacking in myself," Joel explains wistfully. "I became cocky, flip, obstinate, controlling. On-line, I was an animal. That's the therapeutic part. Our soci-ety is not geared toward sexual satisfaction. I came from a strict family. In school I was a potted plant. Then I became a workaholic couch potato. Hypersex saved me. It's like a living Rorschach test. It is more faithful to myself than my unhypered personality is. I saw who I really was; I met myself on-line. Only now I'm a damn cripple. A has-been."

I ask Joel why, now that his hand is shot, he doesn't use a more proper organ for his sexual gratification instead of pining for the Web. Hasn't his Net-therapy given him the confidence to try real sex? "I don't want to go to a Barnes and Noble to make small talk with a stranger and if I get lucky, face the rigors of courtship and seduction," he snaps. "I *am* a recluse. No face-to-face means no embarrassment, no performance anxiety, no emotional risk. I had a noncyber relationship once, but the demands on my time and energy were excessive, the payback small. Cybersex is totally satisfying and a big ego boost. Ninety times out of a hundred its realistic alternative would be no sex at all, or solitary masturbation." People who would not grab a girl's flaunted tits on the street can do so on the Net, which, by virtue of being unreal, doesn't have to espouse established social controls. In the room that it makes for some social acceptance of the desperation and frequency of our sexual needs, the Net is much kinder to our libidos than the real world, and is not, in that narrow sense, unreal.

In his effort to regain a sex life, Joel has invested in Quick-Cam CU-SeeMe software. "Video conferencing offers more identity adjustment than text-chat," he raves. "It lets everyone be film director, makeup artist, set designer, lighting technician, and star. But people are still timid; they leave the camera running on one spot—at best a crotchcam. I talk by mike to get someone's eye-icon to open up. I don't like the sound of my voice, so I use a tape. I had camera sex with a Mauritanian, a Greek, a muscleman in the Urals. I hated it. I like sophisticated illusion. If I push my testicles back, people take it for a beaver shot; if I show my penis, they disconnect." A media fan, Joel knows that the naming, not the being, of a thing draws audience attention. Successful advertising uses adroit words and images that refer to desired immaterialities, which is why there may never be an end to the American dream.

Nowadays the manipulation of images on the Net is abundant. A good example is the Amateur Action BBS in California, an on-line-porn market leader with annual revenues in excess of $1 million that advertises itself as "the nastiest place on earth!" and posts a warning: "Use by law enforcement agents, postal workers and informants is prohibited." Its owner boosts sales by front-loading blurry bucolic pictures explicated as sex with barnyard animals or basic porn scenes described as incest. Images of oral sex are twice as popular when characterized as "choking." Fallacy is in demand, especially if packaged as the naked truth.

Interestingly, the newest craze in the anonymous World Wide Web is self-exposure. The $20-a-month access to the Net that comes with a free Web page has enabled tens of thousands of average Americans to strip for their camera and post a home page with a standard age disclaimer and clickable banners leading to unairbrushed nude shots, dull diary pages, and accounts of sexual feats. Nebraska mothers and Kansas grannies pose nude in their kitchens and backyards and upload the pictures into newsgroups like alt.binaries.pictures.erotica and get more attention than well-directed mating ads on Videodating Connection or doctored images of Hillary Clinton naked before a Nazi flag. Thousands flock to these free amateur pages daily, e-mailing innuendoes, poems, or unsolicited e-gifts, offering thunderous applause for people not attractive or glamorous or outgoing enough to receive notice in the real world. Some like it so much they install video cameras in their bedrooms that feed images of their private lives into their Web pages every three minutes. Those live pages, like Jenni.cam, can get 2 million hits a day, generate discussion groups among fans, and even charge access fees.

Vera is a twenty-six-year-old pear-shaped Memphis Netizen with stringy hair, frightened eyes, prominent teeth, and a drawling accent, a dental hygienist by day and a nude Web star at night. I meet her in a Wendy's, and she breezingly opens up to what she calls my kindred spirit. Wedged into bulging Gap jeans and Gap shirt, Vera looks like a grocery-store checkout girl.

"I've only had two boyfriends," she tells me, "and both called me fat; I never undressed in front of them in the light. My last boyfriend took embarrassing shots of me when I was drunk and posted them on the Net without asking me, to play a joke on me after a fight. And he couldn't believe the hundreds of replies I got. 'You make my blood boil' stuff. I felt humiliated and angry, but I also felt pretty for the first time. I realized I wanted to let go of my hang-ups. He said I was becoming a slut and left me. I didn't care. I bought a tripod and a Canon, took shots, and posted them myself. Now I'm a pro. My family and girlfriends don't use the Net, so it's safe. I now have confidence. I don't want a boyfriend. I had enough of that. I get offers for sex from many fans, but I'm not looking for trouble. Sometimes I masturbate while reading it though." She has never had Net-sex. Her only confidante is her psychic.

Today's Net strikes me as America's version of the ancient Greek agora—the citizens' podium that inevitably turns into their marketplace. Many women flashing their goods for kicks eventually take up grassroots marketing and build strip-product businesses out of their fetishes. With no overhead, no marketing costs, and no suppliers, they can net $50 to $100,000 a year selling their nude calendars or stills and custom videotapes.

It's a safe investment. Media Matrix estimated that 28 percent of Americans visited adult sites in May 1997. Sex searches make up 20 percent of all Web requests. Mom-and-pop virtual sex shops that simply supply sex directories can gross $1 million a year; or they buy CD-ROM X-rated libraries, post them for a fee, and make thousands of dollars a week. Retro-Raunch.com charges members $25 a month to view 5,000 nude pinups dating from 1910 to 1975. Danni's Hard Drive grossed $2.5 million in 1997 by selling $10 monthly memberships to hundreds of photos of nude strippers. Dozens of "stealth sites" designed to confuse the user (WhiteHouse.gov is the site of the White House, WhiteHouse.com is a softporn site) make money each time they get a hit. Small operators also earn thousands of dollars a week carrying advertising for bigger sites—CyberErotica pays a site five cents per customer who clicks on its ads. CyberErotica has 55,000 members and 250,000 daily visitors, offers 10,000 explicit images as well as live videos, erotic audio/text files, and software, and grosses $800,000 a month. An even bigger business is IEG, which plunged its phone-sex profits into live sex video sites and grossed $20 million in 1997. *Playboy* has launched a $7-a-month Cyber Club offering live chats and every Playmate photo, and *Penthouse* plans to create a worldwide Webcam network of video correspondents, using cutting-edge neural and sensory interfaces. These mega–sex merchants are bankrolling innovations like live streaming video and virtual sex, using the proceeds of human sexuality to boost technology.

When Vera got requests for nudes in specific poses or outfits, she acted them out and posted them. Then she saw that other pages offered digital snapshots or audiotapes for $20 to $45 each, and decided to set up a mail-order business; she got a secure line for credit card orders and dealt in panties. "I had so many requests for my panties, I couldn't afford them. So I started charging fifteen dollars a pair; they cost three dollars a pair in bulk, but I won't make my fortune here. I'm not after dirty money. I just like knowing that millions of guys around the world are hot for me and want my intimate things. When I get a hundred e-mails at the end of a day, it's the best thing in my life. I affect millions of people: it's the greatest fulfillment."

Before I flew to Memphis I went on the Net in search of answers to these questions: Could the modem unleash the suspected chaos of human sexuality that entire civilizations have been constructed to restrain? Is America engaging in an open digital revolt against its own sexual repression? Can the Web eventually bridge the fundamental dichotomy that has long set the terms of our carnal existence?

I signed on as Priapus—reasoning that, if I were to go online for sex, I might as well know the fun of inverting myself. My bio preposterously described me as a twenty-seven-year-old MBA, ex–drill sergeant, hairy, dark, 6-foot-3, 210-pound, 10-inch endowed hardbody. Gay submissives and lusty women who I assumed were jaded men sent me instant predatory messages inviting me to private rooms with enticements like "I'm breathing hard," "Cup my 38DDs in your paw," "LAFS—may I drink this Satyr's nectar?" "Swooning in my leather," and, most often, "I ask permission to serve you." No one betrayed any awareness that this wasn't real. Dozens asked me to spank them or feed them my fecal waste, when in fact all they were anxious to do was imagine it.

Jake Baker was a conscientious, introverted University of Michigan sophomore majoring in linguistics who, in 1995, posted alt.sex.stories of kidnapping, sodomizing, and mutilating a real female student; the plot twists involved a ceiling fan, a steel-wire whisk, a spreader bar, a hot curling iron, superglue, and a match. "Torture is foreplay," he wrote, "rape is romance, snuff is climax." When he was charged with transmitting a threat to injure across state lines, he explained that he wanted to be a writer, and that his textual violence was due to his stress over student loans. The charges were dismissed. I now saw why: stories like his cram the electronic rooms and *are* people's sexual contact.

And I noticed that, despite the volume of the sleazy banter daily building an immense X-rated library-in-flux in hundreds of sites named alt.sex.nasalhair, gangbang, alt.sex.snuff.cannibalism, teensex.cum.com, people's revelry follows a uniform linear pattern comparable to a mechanical barter of goods

("How big are your tits?" "How big is your dick?"). Most fornicators exchange prosaic back-and-forth descriptions of what they are doing to each other in regurgitations of *Penthouse* Forum clichés laden with emoticons and acronyms. The sex act is a series of lines such as "Spreading your legs," "Making me wet," "Rubbing your thighs," "Wiggling hips." Net-sex proved to me that interconnectedness doesn't necessarily foster originality. At best, Net-sex is a purging of passions, of value only as a secularized confessional.

I soon learned that Netiquette obliged me to be screenally assaulted by impertinent, uninvited bellows in overlapping boxes flashing their raw need to be heard; horny, invisible men crashed my system, delayed my other mail, unloaded oceans of gruesome particulars into my nervous cortex, and stalked me with unsigned exultant missives like "Hot now do me LO." I did not feel wanted. I felt pummeled like a scapegoat. Priapus retired, and I was exhilarated to be free of all his agitated cyberwooers.

Feeling somewhat traumatized by cyberlust, I became curious about its real repercussions. I found the Net is equally full of angry discussions of ruined marriages, gender dysfunction, personality dichotomy, stalking, rape, murder. In August 1997, the American Psychological Association's meeting in Chicago focused on the "dangers of seeking love on-line" and its links to escalating clinical depression. But the most common Net-affliction is addiction. The new Internet addiction disorder damages children's and teens' lives and costs adults their families, friendships, and jobs, according to Kimberly Young, author of *Caught in the Net: How to Recognize the Signs of Internet Addiction.* Young estimates 5 to 17 percent of users are addicts. The heavy users Young interviewed log on to escape problems and cheer up, then need increasing on-line time to attain satisfaction and feel irritable if they try to curb the habit. Fifty-two percent are in recovery programs for other addictions and are using the Net instead of alcohol, gambling, or drugs; 54 percent have a history of depression. Psychiatrist Ivan Goldberg, who coined the IAD term, believes the Net can be an avoidance tool for distressed individuals; Goldberg prescribes antidepressants to his clients who can't regulate their time on-line.

Martha is a self-employed Memphis pharmacist I meet through abstruse Net-chat routes, the mother of two undergraduates, happily married for twenty-two years to a successful pharmacologist. She has a round, drowsy face, nimble posture, pillowy behind, and is wearing a pink CP Shades outfit and matching beret. She takes me to the mall for a Wolfgang Puck pizza and confides that a cyberaffair was the "big wake-up call" in her quiet life.

She got into cyberinfidelity out of ignorance. "I had no idea what I was getting into, since I never had a desire to look at another man during my marriage. My husband didn't mind: it stayed on the Net; he saw it like my reading a *Playgirl*. It didn't seem real, so I couldn't see why I was getting so involved. I became emotionally dependent on the typed words. First the courtship ritual seduced me. I got unfettered attention, soulmating, dreamy romance. It all seemed refreshingly orderly, dignified. I liked the intimacy men were expressing that my husband didn't and compared them to the imperfect man I knew at home. I saw that people in the rest of the world could be entranced by my words. And I had the most exciting sex I ever experienced. I got hooked; my phone was always tied up, I neglected my family, my job, my social life, the outdoors; I only thought about the next time I could link on. I'd make love with my husband and then go on-line for more and I'd be so giddy I couldn't sleep. The Net was my second home. The safety of being in my home allowed me to be free of the white lies and half-truths of everyday life. All the tangible messy real-life stuff fell away, I was nervy and frank and narcissistic, and I needed it like a narcotic," she confesses soberly. I understand Net-sex provides a welcome equilibrium to a mind agitated by daily preoccupations; by opening up an unequivocal parenthesis of relaxation and narcosis (the space of a Borgesian dream—a dream that can be entered into by other people also dreaming), it functions as a blockage to the outside world. It's a reality antidote.

"I know it's real sex," Martha warns me sternly, "because the repercussions are real. The Net tore up our family. My husband moved out. I didn't want to lose him so I stopped my on-line affair, but I felt like I'd died. I never had any partner except my husband in my life before this. There's a dangerous temptation to treat cybersex as a sedative, or a game, as if we're interacting with an artificial intelligence. Our society has no established mores about cybersex. The government should educate the public and address this issue, not just urge us to get computer-literate. It's time to start worrying."

"The Net is re-creating the sixties," Virgil says, crossing his white-Armani-trousered legs with tactful, territorial aggression, "at a time when, because of AIDS, hepatitis B, and all, indiscriminate anonymous sex can't happen in the real world, and everyone warns us against too much sex." We're in his wood-paneled office on the top floor of a Disney-esque castle with ivied tapered turrets blatantly designed to evoke the *idea* of a northeastern educational Elysium. I'm thinking that so much of modernity is only the superifcial, jazzed-up reinvention of seasoned wisdoms and techniques whose essence may be irredeemably lost.

Virgil looks at me as if I were a gathering storm. He still looks afraid of himself, menaced by his own excited blood. "We're scared to sleep together," he suddenly adds. "The Net would have eliminated that." Because it would keep us isolated, I say. "You're always either eluding or quoting," he answers in melancholic resignation. "I doubt I've heard you say a single authentic line." In former ages, I tell him, there was no separation between the most abstract forms of thinking and the most sensual forms of erotic pleasure; they usually happened in tandem. Why can't we discuss the Net, quote Epicurus, and fuck? He stares at me in stupified silence. I sense a moment of greater epiphany here: he's come around to my point of view. Neither one of us knows how to act freely. We've said too much, done too little. We sit across from each other, touchable and puzzled and preoccupied, and for this we can't forgive ourselves. In a sense, we remain two screens. We can't get face-to-face.

"At least we can talk of sex freely," Virgil points out. "Our parents couldn't do that. Net-sex teaches us to say what we like. We wouldn't be sitting here, two people so different and so alike, if it weren't for that." I say that each technological improvement to which we adapt takes us a step farther from our genetic selves rooted in the past, as we're trading experience for abbreviation and confinement; cyberspace makes us even more withdrawn, sphinxlike ghosts pared into pure information. He bridles in his swivel chair. "Cybersex is a legitimate release for people who can't get it otherwise," he insists. "It can't satiate the soul, but that's life: I thought you and I were so soulful, and look at us now." I disagree: Net-talk obsesses with physical description precisely because the absence of the sexual body is troubling us. That's what leaves us fundamentally unsatisfied. Cyberpleasure is tinged with our absence.

"At least on the Net I had hygienic, discreet sex without physically cheating on my wife or endangering her with my extracurricular activities, or feeling the debilitating frustration and sickening terror I feel next to you now," Virgil rebuts. "If you must know the truth, the instant I saw you, I thought 'Here comes trouble!' I'm not up for so much emotion; I feel exhausted, drained. So I guess I'd rather stay on-line and have peace. I call it creative adultery. I'm married, but my cyberself does not have to be."

"What distinguishes man from animals," Anatole France

wrote, "is lying and literature." I had thought Net-sex might well be an accurate litmus test of the American libido. I now know that what goes on in people's minds does not reflect what goes on in their beds. The fact is, most of us basically want a home, a mate, a stable life; and from time to time we also want to be everything: architects of destruction, lumberjacks, gypsies, heartbreakers, violators and violated. The Net is the most abstract satisfaction of our most concrete desire to appropriate, and possess, the world. The unnerving irony is that people can be as uncivilized as they're naturally inclined to be only with the help of an ur-civilized technology that reduces sex to a disembodied, vaporous transgression. Static torpor disguised as frenetic interactivity is the medium's actual magnetism. Cybersex is about our ingrained fear of sex and our self-exiling fear of the body. In response, Virgil, looking both courtly and sodden, starts to recite "The Love Song of J. Alfred Prufrock"; by the time he reaches the part about the hundred indecisions and hundred visions and revisions, right before he gets to ask " 'Do I dare?' and 'Do I dare?' " I ask him to drive me to the hotel.

That night I watch on my hotel TV Howard Stern reporting jovially behind his permed maenadic tresses that he just had the best blow job of his life with a sex robot prototype he was asked to sample. The newest "sexbots" sport human features in pliant latex, vibrators for tactile stimulation, sound systems for love talk. They are disease-free, nonjudgmental, always aroused. A university professor writing in the August 1997 issue of the *Futurist* I'm reading, predicts that robotic sex will "reduce teen pregnancy, STDs, abortions, pedophilia, and prostitution." He allows for sexbot-related afflictions like addiction and technovirgins ("humans who will never have sex with other humans or even desire it"), but concludes: "Robotic sex may be better than human sex. Like many other technologies that have replaced human endeavors, robots may surpass human technique; because they would be programmable, sexbots would meet each individual user's needs." In the same issue of the *Futurist*, two professors of biology look forward to the day when "odors, tastes, touch, pressure, and kinesthetic sensations" will be bioelectronically reproducible. "Virtual sex will greatly enhance normal sensations," they write, "and add some never before experienced. . . . Virtual sex for the first time will allow safe prostitution and safe sex. Virtual sex will be preferred to surreptitious affairs, cocktail bar pickups. . . . Advanced devices will stimulate the specific pleasure centers of the brain to enhance sensations beyond anything experienced naturally." I note how thoroughly we have adopted the idea that sex is unsafe, and an unscrupulous indistinction between virtual and real; the assumption that virtual is better than real may be our era's most important philosophical shift. "The world of sex is at the threshold of trends amounting to a 21st-century revolution, bringing about the most dramatic changes in sexual relationships, habits, health, pleasures, pains . . . [that] the world has ever seen," the article concludes. I may not be at risk of preferring Net-sex in a phantom zone or supersonic sex with an image I watch on TV to the unscriptable mating dance with a clear-eyed stranger in a sawdust bar, but I can't shake a premonition that my descendants may never know the difference. If sexual technological enhancements affect our erotic subtlety as much as computers already affect our long-distance sight, discos our hearing, preservatives our taste buds, our descendants may never know that the body is infinitely richer than the machine. And there is nothing we can or want to do about this because the process of innovation itself is so enticing and empowering, and snowballing. Novelty, even forgery, has become sublimely sexy.

Memphis on a spring Sunday has a quiet dignity. In the low-rise downtown, strangers smile at me. Everything seems to be rising: odors, cries, songs, horns, birds, water-sprinkled greens, lilac blues. It's a world in idle suspense, unfinished and pregnant with infinity. I'm savoring the slow spill of the sunset, contemplating how easy it has been for me to leave Virgil, click him off, cyberman that he was. As my gaze travels over sunbeams, bodies, houses, cars, windowpanes, I suddenly stretch out my arms as if I were meaning to fly, and an elemental force seems to explode from me and fling me into the rambling crowd.

A Postscript

"Still deeper the meaning of that story of Narcissus, who because he could not grasp the tormenting, mild image he saw in the fountain, plunged into it and was drowned. But that same image, we ourselves see. . . . It is the image of the ungraspable phantom of life; and this is the key to it all."

Herman Melville, Moby Dick

"I think I will do nothing for a long time but listen,
And accrue what I hear into myself . . . and let sounds contribute toward me.

I too am not a bit tamed . . . I too am untranslatable,
I sound my barbaric yawp over the roofs of the world."

Walt Whitman, Leaves of Grass

"As I was saying listening to repeating is often irritating, always repeating is all of living, everything in a being is always repeating, more and more listening to repeating gives to me complete understanding. Each one slowly comes to be a whole one to me. Each one slowly comes to be a whole one in me. . . . Many things then come out in the repeating that make a history of each one for any one who always listens to them. Many things come out of each one and as one listens to them, listens to all the repeating in them, always this comes to be clear about them, the history of them, of the bottom nature in them, the nature or natures mixed up in them to make the whole. . . ."

Gertrude Stein, The Making of Americans

I love you": three ambiguous, impregnable, overused words. Yet they keep fear at bay. They convince us we're good, essential, vital. They suggest the promised land is here, in the fragile region of our own bodies. They give us our humanity, our mysticism, our confidence, our hope. They say we don't have to be like Sisyphus. They say there is more to us than us.

"The first requisite for a gentleman," Nietzsche said, "is to be a perfect animal." Our animal bodies are our common denominator, our meeting point, our link to the greater life around, before, and behind us. Without them, our arrogance would be boundless, our isolation unbearable. Our bodies are not merely the violated forms conjured up in the nightly news, or the titillating shapes exhibited on billboards and city buses, or the perishable mechanisms whose upkeep requires work-outs, massages, deprivations, and healthisms of all kinds. The fact that so many Americans today fault their bodies for their unhappiness does not prove that the primary flaw of our human condition is our bodies that are imperfect; we have learned to base our human uniqueness on our analytical intelligence, so we blame our sense of displacement, anonymity, or abjection on our genetic frailty and turn to technology for help. But in place of desire, we feel unease. Instead of gratification, we find addiction. Rather than awe, we face inconsequence. And despite all our free talk, we feel little secure and at home in our overinterpreted world. Worse still, in our search for finite answers, we become self-exploited, getting our kicks from watching and hearing each other's sexual slips. This may be the apogee of our repression, a puritanism pared down to its naked core: public voyeurism enacted with impunity. The overwhelming pervasiveness of sex as the central issue in our public life over the past decade, in congressional hearings, epic criminal trials, interminable scandals, in our entertain-ment, our habits of consumption, daily life, points to the utter bafflement over what is public and what private, what right and what wrong, to a culture in moral flux. Our confusion saps our courage—the courage it would take for the president of the United States to tell the clamoring cameras he will not testify in public about his personal life because what happens in his bedroom is between him and those he sleeps with and his God; even the puny courage it takes for me to change my mind this late: I now think the cause of our sexual crisis is not the cultural mind-set that locates pleasure in idealized perfection (emphasizing "perfect" over "animal"), and not our lack of wholeness or backbone or activism or knowledge; it is the depletion of our inherent respect for what is unfamiliar, dangerous, and undefined in our nature, our "failure" to love all that we can't control; which is the only love we can reasonably signify when we say to another: "I love you."

This was what I was thinking when I left Memphis. I finally felt ready to begin my actual road trip. I could now embark on it with a fresh and lucid attitude of enlightened wonder. By this or that coincidence I had accumulated a thousand pages of transcribed interviews and I knew something premeditated had to happen to all that material now. My verbatim transcripts didn't read real to me who knew the difference by having been there. I didn't go back to New York, where the phone was bound to ring and send me off on another adventure, but decided to drive across the country, stopping at gas stations and bars and diners and motels and talking to people, filling up my time with gauzy ephemera, so I could discover and test my ideas by my senses. I would casually bring up S/M, priests, strip clubs, cross-dressers, Don Juan, military sex, the Web, and strangers would tell me stories. Those stories would give the third dimension to my skeletal grid and help me fill it out by committing a necessary fraud: splicing together the transcripts I had with the testimonies I got on the road. And then I would do my penance and write the book, alone at a remote spot with hundreds and hundreds of disparate details to melt together into an amalgam of my experiences and the lives at the very end of my reach. Unless another coincidence, or a string of them, derailed me again. And because of the abundance that is the beauty of America, and because the realm of the body is limitless, I had an uncanny hunch that I might never finish this book. I still wasn't even convinced I could write it, or anyone could, even as everyone seemed to want to.

But I already felt satisfied because I had by now come to appreciate the value of what theologians call "wise ignorance": the willingness to acknowledge that what we know increasingly reveals what we don't know. I had expected to bring some of our secrets to light and, by so doing, take away their power to intimidate. Instead, I found not the darkness stirring behind the normalcy of America, but the normalcy stirring peacefully behind the darkness. Rather than penetrating the civilized surface of everyday life to reveal the passions seething under picket-fence respectabilities, I uncovered a robust, unruffled normality plodding beneath these Americans' skin-deep, self-determined perversions. Most of all, I learned that people's desire for originality grew out of a deeper, less hip need for continuity and safety and uniformity—and love.

Notes

Guys as Dolls

24 *15 million* Peggy Rudd, *My Husband Wears My Clothes* (Katy, Texas: PM Publishers, 1989), p. 115.

24 *3 to 5 percent of the male population* Susan Crain Bakos, *Kink: The Hidden Sex Lives of Americans* (New York: St. Martin's Press, 1995), p. 242.

24 Journal of the American Psychoanalytic Association . . . *it relives "enfemme"* Rudd, op. cit., pp. 111–112 and 131–134.

36 *role models* Leslie Feinberg, *Transgender Warriors: From Joan of Arc to RuPaul* (Boston: Beacon Press, 1996).

43 *the week's* Newsweek Daniel Pedersen, "Crossing Over," *Newsweek*, 4 November 1996, p. 66.

43 *a picture of myself* Louise Rafkin, "Conventional Cross-Dressers," *Out*, February 1997, p. 27.

Masters of Ceremony

49 *S/Ms are mostly men . . . ten to one* Susan Crain Bakos, *Kink: The Hidden Sex Lives of Americans* (New York: St. Martin's Press, 1995), pp. 57–58.

51 *AIDS is credited . . . "as long as nobody gets hurt"* Ibid., pp. xvii and xx.

51 *Forced sex . . . The Kinsey Institute . . . regularly* Ibid., p. xix.

57 *PONY . . . reports* Ibid., p. xix.

War in Peace

69 *two out of three . . . largest day-care provider* John Barry and Evan Thomas, "At War Over Women," *Newsweek*, 12 May 1997, p. 48.

69–70 *William Kite . . . statements . . . on his base* Elaine Sciolino, "Courtship Leads to Marriage and Maybe Officer's Ouster," *The New York Times*, 3 July 1997.

70 *sailors aboard the . . .* Nimitz John Barry and Evan Thomas, "Shifting Lines," *Newsweek*, 16 June 1997, p. 31.

71 *Lt. Kelly Flinn . . . modern wars* Gregory Vistica and Evan Thomas, "Sex and Lies," *Newsweek*, 2 June 1997, pp. 27–31; Roger Angell, "Sins Like Flinn's," *The New Yorker*, 2 June 1997, p. 5.

72 *the 1991 Tailhook convention scandal . . . resigned* Peter J. Boyer,

"Admiral Boorda's War," *The New Yorker,* 16 September 1996, pp. 71–72.

72 *The suicide of Navy Chief* Ibid., p. 71.

73 *the words of Navy secretary J. D. Howard* Ibid., p. 84.

73 *Because of Tailhook, Congresswoman Pat Schroeder . . . bill* Ibid., p. 72.

74 *8 percent of America's new coed force . . . pregnant* Stephanie Gutmann, "Sex and the Soldier," *The New Republic,* 24 February 1997, p. 21.

74 *In the Gulf War, 39 of the 400 . . . "hell tours"* Barry and Thomas, "At War Over Women," *Newsweek,* 12 May 1997, p. 48; Gutmann, "Sex and the Soldier," p. 22.

74 *Women make up 14 percent . . . 20 to 25 percent of new recruits* Mark Thompson, "Offensive Maneuvers," *Time,* 5 May 1997, p. 42; Barry and Thomas, *Newsweek,* 12 May 1997, p. 48.

74 *Since 1994 . . . eighty thousand jobs . . . combat ships* The New York Times, 3 July 1997, p. A1.

74 *recruiters lower the official standards* Gutmann, "Sex and the Soldier," p. 19.

74 *Staff Sgt. Delmar Simpson . . . went AWOL* Elaine Sciolino, "The Army's Problems with Sex and Power," *The New York Times,* 5 May 1997; Jamie McIntyre, "Aberdeen Commander Suspended," *U.S. News & World Report,* 2 July 1997; Gregory Vistica, "War in the Ranks," *Newsweek,* 25 November 1996, pp. 29–31; Elizabeth Gleick, "Scandal in the Military," *Time,* 25 November 1996, pp. 28–31.

75 *the victims' courtroom testimonies . . . respect* Sciolino, op. cit., 5 May 1997.

75 *80 percent of the victims . . . accused black* Gleick, "Scandal in the Military," p. 30.

75–76 *Sgt. Maj. Gene McKinney . . . fifty-six years in prison* Gregory Vistica and Evan Thomas, "Trouble in the Ranks," *Newsweek,* 17 February 1997, pp. 46–47; Henry Louis Gates Jr., "Men Behaving Badly," *The New Yorker,* 18 August 1997, pp. 4–5.

76 *"the Army's dirty laundry"* Associated Press, "Attorney May Air Dirty Laundry," *The New York Times,* 13 August 1997.

76 *Cmdr. Robert Davis . . . Laughton, of racism* Evan Thomas and Gregory Vistica, "At War in the Ranks," *Newsweek,* 11 August 1997, pp. 32–33.

76 *Capt. Everett Greene . . . career* Ibid., p. 32.

76–77 *thousands . . . every year . . . ten times more often* Vistica, op. cit., p. 30.

77 *Confidential Army case . . . gunpoint* Ibid., p. 30.

77 *Pentagon surveys . . . sexual harassment* Barry and Thomas, *Newsweek,* 12 May 1997, p. 49.

77 *September 1997, the Army released its largest study . . . overseeing moral training* Associated Press, "Army: Sexual Harassment Is Rampant," *The New York Times,* 11 September 1997.

77 *November 1996 . . . sexual harassment hot line . . . Fort Sam Houston medic school* Vistica, op. cit., p. 30.

77–78 *Veterans Administration study . . . battle trauma* Ibid., p. 31; Gleick, "Scandal in the Military," p. 28.

78 *during the Gulf War . . . knifepoint by a sergeant* Gutmann, "Sex and the Soldier," p. 22.

78 *"We relaxed . . . Gen. Dennis Reimer . . . we can"* John Barry, "At War in the Barracks," *Newsweek*, 17 February 1997, p. 47.

78 *In June 1995, two SEAL buddies . . . vaginas* Maximillian Potter, "Her Fate Was Sealed," *Details*, May 1997, pp. 186–193.

79 *in September 1995 . . . on Okinawa . . . Richard Macke . . . cost him his job* Boyer, "Admiral Boorda's War," p. 85.

84 *In June 1997, Air Force general Joseph Ralston . . . of Flinn's case* John Barry and Evan Thomas, "Shifting Lines," *Newsweek*, 16 June 1997, pp. 28–30.

84 *Ralston had signed . . . Lt. Gen. Thomas Griffith . . . conference* Ibid., p. 30.

85 *average woman has less height . . . pee standing up in the field* Barry and Thomas, *Newsweek*, 12 May 1997, p. 49; Gutmann, "Sex and the Soldier," p. 20.

85 *every aviator . . . "clearance scrub"* Boyer, "Admiral Boorda's War," p. 83.

87 *Until the seventies . . . "Rape, kill, mutilate"* Barbara Ehrenreich, "Wartime in the Barracks," *Time*, 2 December 1996, p. 96.

Blood Simple Babes

93–94 *The local papers . . . hairdos* More on this in Andrea Juno, and V. Vale, eds., *Modern Primitives* (San Francisco: RE/Search Publications, 1989).

106 *Dr. Paul MacLean . . . sexual excitement* Michael Segell, "Make Love and War," *Esquire*, August 1997, p. 98.

107 Newsweek-*reported poll* Michele Ingrassia, "Body of the Beholder," *Newsweek*, 24 April 1995, pp. 66–67.

107 *Raelyn Gallina* Marilee Strong, "A Bright Red Scream," *San Francisco Focus*, November 1993, pp. 138–39.

111–12 *Different psychiatrists . . . illness, or injury* Ibid., pp. 59, 60, 64, 65, and 136.

112 *In a six-month study . . . UCSF . . . cutting* Ibid., p. 135.

112 *An estimated 2 million* Ibid., p. 59.

112–13 *Favazza . . . fifty times* Ibid., p. 63.

113 *Self-Mutilators Anonymous (SMA) . . . SAFE* Ibid., p. 63.

113 *SIV . . . stigma* Ibid., p. 60.

The Economy of Desire

118 *Michael J. Peters . . . in 1982* *Exotic Dancer Bulletin*, no. 1, Spring 1996, p. 10.

118 U.S. News & World Report . . . *1987* Eric Schlosser, "The Business

of Pornography," *U.S. News & World Report,* 10 February 1997, pp. 42–50.

119 *"Lifestyles of the Rich and Famous"* . . .Allure   Cabaret Royale promotional material.

119–20 *By the end of the eighties . . . back-wage liabilities*   Exotic Dancer Bulletin, no. 1, Spring 1996, pp. 13–15.

Intercourse by Numbers

137 The Cincinnatian   *The Cincinnatian,* January/February 1995.

149 *Sex and Love*   SLAA pamphlet (Boston: The Augustine Fellowship, 1995).

149 *twelve hundred SAA groups meeting*   SAA pamphlet (Minneapolis: National Service Organization of SAA, 1995).

153 *Carnes estimates that 3 to 6 percent*   Karen Garloch, "Experts Differ on Whether Certain Sexual Behaviors Are True Illnesses," Knight Ridder Newspapers, 6 October 1998.

153 *research shows . . . education*   Abraham Verghese, "Annals of Addiction," *The New Yorker,* 16 February 1998, p. 47.

153 *Their preoccupation with . . . compulsion*   Liane Evans, "Interview with Patrick Carnes: Don't Call It Love," *The Northeast Recovery Networker,* November 1994, p. 7.

152 *"Harold C. Lyon"* . . . Washington Post,   *Out of the Shadows: Understanding Sexual Addiction* (Minneapolis: National Service Organization of SAA, 1995), p. 133.

154 *"James Cermak's attorney"*   Ibid., p. 63.

154–55 *According to Carnes . . . sixty of them*   Evans, op. cit., p. 6.

155 *"Forty Questions for Self-Diagnosis"*   SLAA pamphlet (Boston: The Augustine Fellowship, 1995).

Virgins at Heart

164 *10 percent of American priests . . . to marry*   Richard Sipe, *Sex, Priests, and Power: Anatomy of a Crisis* (New York: Brunner/Mazzel, 1995), p. 120.

165 *80 percent . . . masturbate*   Ibid., p. 70.

163–64 *half the American clergy favor . . . to marry*   Jason Berry, *Lead Us Not into Temptation: Catholic Priests and the Sexual Abuse of Children* (New York: Image Books, Doubleday Press, 1992), p. 174.

164 *America's Catholic population . . . by 80 percent*   Ibid., pp. 173 and 259.

164 *Association of Catholic Priests . . . service*   Sipe, op. cit., p. 121.

164–65 *2 percent of Catholic priests . . . homosexual*   Ibid., pp. ix and 27; Berry, op. cit., pp. xx, 186, 187, 188, and 213.

165 *1982 to 1992 . . . adults*   Berry, p. ixx.

180 *$500 million in official losses . . . for sexual crimes*   Ibid., pp. ixx, 99, and 279.

180 *Victims of Clergy Abuse (LINKUP)*   Sipe, op. cit., p. 37.

Tales from the Crypt

186–87 *"Sexual Attraction . . . to corpses"* J. P. Rosman and P. J. Resnick, "Sexual Attraction to Corpses: A Psychiatric Review of Necrophilia," *Bulletin of the American Academy of Psychiatry and the Law* 17, no. 2 (1989), pp. 153–163.

187–88 *She said she had . . . "men in their twenties"* Jim Morton, "The Unrepentant Necrophile: An Interview with Karen Greenlee," *Apocalypse Culture* (Portland: Feral House, 1990), pp. 28–35.

Alien Romance

199 *Barney and Betty Hill* J. G. Fuller, *The Interrupted Journey* (New York: Dial Press, 1966).

199 *1 percent . . . 2.25 million* C. D. B. Bryan, *Close Encounters of the Fourth Kind: A Reporter's Notebook on Alien Abduction, UFOs, and the Conference at M.I.T.* (New York: Arkana, Penguin Books, 1995), p. 235.

199 *560,000 and 3.7 million* Randall Rothenberg, "Area 51, Where Are You?" *Esquire*, September 1996, p. 93.

199 *A 1991 Roper poll* John Mack, *Abduction: Human Encounters with Aliens* (New York: Charles Scribner's Sons, 1994), p. 448.

200 *1992 MIT abduction conference . . . twenty-first century* Andrea Pritchard, David Pritchard, John Mack, Pam Kasey, and Claudia Yapp, eds., *Alien Discussions: Proceedings of the Abduction Study Conference* (Cambridge, Massachusetts: North Cambridge Press, 1995).

200 *Like most . . . to UFO lore* Bryan, op. cit., p. 7.

201 *Dr. Jacobs interviewed . . . removed* David Jacobs, *Secret Life: First-hand Accounts of UFO Abductions* (New York: Simon & Schuster, 1992); Bryan, op. cit., pp. 19 and 26.

201 *Budd Hopkins . . . fifteen hundred cases . . . raped* Bryan, op. cit., p. 33.

205–6 *Dr. Richard Boylan . . . defeat them* Ibid., pp. 129 and 165–181.

206 *49 percent of all Americans believe* Harper's Index, *Harper's*, December 1996, p. 13.

206 *John Lear* Rothenberg, op. cit., p. 94.

206–7 *Recent experiments . . . vulnerable to them* Bryan, op. cit., pp. 438 and 440–441.

213 *Some psychiatrists . . . ritual abuse* Ibid., p. 138.

215 *Raelian cult* Zed Frick, "God Rides a UFO: Interview with Rael's New York representative, David Uzal," *Cups*, May 1996, pp. 6–8.

Hypercoitus

226 *Sharon Lopatka and Robert Glass* "Death on the Internet," *Time*, 18 November 1996, p. 104.

228 *Hot chat was launched . . . e-rooms* Jeff Goodell, "The Fevered Rise of America Online," *Rolling Stone*, 3 October 1996, p. 61.

228 *By 1996 . . . $7 million a month* Ibid., pp. 60 and 64.

228 *Love at AOL . . . a month* Marilyn Elias, "Online Is a Loveline for Many," *USA Today*, 14 August 1997.

228–29 *of the 35 to 40*   Goodell, op. cit., p. 62.

229 *A 1995 Carnegie Mellon . . . networks*   Philip Elmer-Dewitt, "On a Screen Near Your: Cyberporn," *Time*, 3 July 1995, pp. 38–45.

231 *Experts estimate that two . . . men*   Elias, op. cit.

232 *Oliver Jovanovic*   Linda Wolfe, "Attorney for the Offense," *New York*, 2 March 1998.

235 *Amateur Action BBS*   Wendy Cole, "The Marquis de Cyberspace," *Time*, 3 July 1995, pp. 46–47.

236–37 *Media Matrix estimated . . . sensory interfaces*   Vic Sussman, "Sex Sites Hot on the Web," *USA Today*, 22 August 1997.

238 *Jake Baker . . . loans*   Philip Elmer-Dewitt, "Snuff Porn on the Net," *Time*, 20 February 1995, p. 69.

239 *In August 1997, the American . . . depression*   Elias, op. cit.

239 *Kimberly Young . . . on-line time*   Marilyn Elias and Elizabeth Wiese, "Digital Drug," *USA Today*, 15 April 1998.

243–44 *A university professor writing . . . needs"*   Kenneth Maxwell, "Sex in the Future: Virtuous and Virtual?" *The Futurist*, July/August 1997, pp. 29–31; Joel Snell, "Impacts of Robotic Sex," *The Futurist*, July/August 1997, p. 32.

244 *In the same issue of the* Futurist *. . . has ever seen"*   Marvin Cetron and Owen Davies, "Smart Toasters, Media Butlers, and More," *The Futurist*, July/August 1997, pp. 19–23.